ISSUES IN NURSING RESEARCH

ISSUES
IN
NURSING
RESEARCH

Florence S. Downs, R.N., Ed.D., F.A.A.N.
Associate Dean, Graduate Education
University of Pennsylvania
School of Nursing
Philadelphia, Pennsylvania

Juanita W. Fleming, R.N., Ph.D., F.A.A.N.
Assistant Dean for Graduate Education
Director of Graduate Studies
College of Nursing
Health Science Learning Center
University of Kentucky
Lexington, Kentucky

APPLETON-CENTURY-CROFTS/New York

79 80 81 82 83 / 10 9 8 7 6 5 4 3 2 1

Prentice-Hall International, Inc., London
Prentice-Hall of Australia, Pty. Ltd., Sydney
Prentice-Hall of India Private Limited, New Delhi
Prentice-Hall of Japan, Inc., Tokyo
Prentice-Hall of Southeast Asia (Pte.) Ltd., Singapore
Whitehall Books Ltd., Wellington, New Zealand

Library of Congress Cataloging in Publication Data

Downs, Florence S
  Issues in nursing research.

  Includes index.
  1. Nursing—Research. I. Fleming, Juanita W., joint
author. II. Cleland, Virginia S. III. Title.
RT81.5.D67   610.73′072   78-21914
ISBN 0-8385-4436-3

Text design: Laurie Wilkowski
Cover design: Karin Batten

PRINTED IN THE UNITED STATES OF AMERICA

CONTRIBUTORS

Virginia S. Cleland, R.N., Ph.D., F.A.A.N.
Professor
College of Nursing
Wayne State University
Detroit, Michigan

Florence S. Downs, R.N., Ed.D., F.A.A.N.
Associate Dean, Graduate Education
University of Pennsylvania
School of Nursing
Philadelphia, Pennsylvania

Juanita W. Fleming, R.N., Ph.D., F.A.A.N.
Assistant Dean for Graduate Education
Director of Graduate Studies
College of Nursing
Health Science Learning Center
University of Kentucky
Lexington, Kentucky

Susan Gortner, M.N., Ph.D., F.A.A.N.
Associate Dean for Research
School of Nursing
University of California at San Francisco
San Francisco, California

Jean Hayter, R.N., Ed.D., F.A.A.N.
Professor
College of Nursing
University of Kentucky
Lexington, Kentucky

Joanne S. Stevenson, R.N., Ph.D., F.A.A.N
Associate Professor and Assistant Director for Research
Director
Center for Nursing Research
The Ohio State University School of Nursing
Columbus, Ohio

Carolyn A. Williams, R.N., Ph.D., F.A.A.N.
Associate Professor
School of Nursing
Assistant Professor of Epidemiology
School of Allied Health
University of North Carolina
Chapel Hill, North Carolina

CONTENTS

PREFACE

This volume has been prepared with a full understanding that there is a diversity of opinion regarding the nature of research in nursing and what constitutes the most valid means to accomplish the expansion of nursing knowledge. However, beneath this diversity lies a common concern for improving the quality of the nursing process as a means for enhancing the health of people. We believe that an appreciation of the issues surrounding the research process is in the interest of promoting this conviction. We also believe that greater insight into the complexity of the decisions that must be made relative to research activity can help to create an atmosphere more conducive to and supportive of research in nursing.

This book is intended for consumers of nursing research, researchers, educators, administrators, and particularly graduate students who wish to pinpoint some of the problematic areas encountered on the way to research implementation. We are convinced that the issues we have chosen to address lie close to the heart of the research process, and that it is unlikely that they will be resolved in the near future. Yet each reader may need to work through them at some time on the basis of their personal predilections.

We have made every effort to enlist authors who are authorities on and vitally interested in the particular problem addressed. We begin with an overview of the trends in nursing research and then progress to a look at the future. Each chapter can stand alone in the contribution it makes or be weighed in relation to the others.

We are grateful for the patience and support of our editor, Charles Bollinger.

ISSUES
IN
NURSING
RESEARCH

CHAPTER ONE

TRENDS AND HISTORICAL PERSPECTIVE

Susan Gortner

As the nation enters the final quarter of this century, nursing is moving toward a more prominent and responsible position on the health scene than it has held in the past. The extent to which nursing can exert social influence through its particular body of knowledge and skills is a function of (a) the competence of its practitioners, scholars, and new recruits; (b) the capacity it may have to bring about positive results in the health status of its clientele; and (c) the continued appraisal and extension of that capacity through basic and clinical research, as well as through the activities of related health fields.

The conduct of its own research, together with a small nucleus of well-prepared investigators, represents a recent phenomenon for nursing. Most notably this has occurred in the last 15 or 20 years, although the antecedents of nursing research go back over 100 years to Miss Nightingale herself. In this chapter an attempt will be made to first document the more recent trends in nursing research activity and development, and then to provide an historical perspective against which the reader may want to reflect our present state. The author's perspective is drawn from ten years' association with national programs of federal grants and contracts to support nursing research, and to support nurse fellows undergoing research training in nursing and in the substantive fields basic to nursing. While these programs do not represent the entire universe of research activity in nursing, the fact that they are nationwide and, for the most part, investigator initiated allows them to serve as barometers of current and future directions. It should be remembered that

1

the field is relatively young and its nurse investigators are still of the first generation. Against this backdrop, the past decade or two reveal noteworthy accomplishments.

RECENT TRENDS

The Bicentennial Year represented a milestone of sorts for the growing field of nursing research, and for the growing body of nurses who are interested in using the tools of research to improve the general health of the population. In no previous time in the historical development of research in this country has there been as much interest in research activities in nursing, especially in the areas of research related to practice.[1] In addition to this interest, the United States is in the enviable position of having the largest number of nurses prepared in research in the world. The latest figures are being updated, but the estimate is over 1,800 for nurses with earned doctorates in the United States, with the most significant increase in numbers occurring within the last five years.

Passage of Public Law 94-278 in April 1976 authorized amendments to the National Research Service Act of 1974 to include the research and research training programs of the Division of Nursing, United States Public Health Service (USPHS). After a three-year hiatus, applications for nurse predoctoral and postdoctoral research fellowships could thus be solicited and the preparation of future scientific talent assured. In September of 1976, the prestigious special committee of the National Academy of Sciences, charged under the 1974 Act with establishing the nation's need for biomedical and behavioral research personnel, for the first time took up consideration of nursing research areas and research training needs in its continued study of scientific talent.* The 94th Congress specified $5,000,000 for research projects in nursing, and $1,000,000 for research fellowships to be spent during the 1977 and 1978 fiscal years, with particular attention to those studies that would improve the quality and delivery of nursing care. These figures represent the first earmarking of funds for nursing research in the appropriation. Research studies figured prominently in the major programs of the American Nurses' Association Biennial Conventions in Atlantic City and Honolulu. The Commission on Nursing Research of that organization has presented research programs that were very well attended and has prepared a number of publications for both the public and the profession on the nature of nursing research,

---

*It was the author's privilege to speak on behalf of the field and the federal effort at this meeting. The Committee's 1977 Report, entitled *Personnel Needs and Training for Biomedical and Behavioral Research* devoted an entire chapter to nursing research.

research priorities in nursing, preparation of the nurse researcher and ethical guidelines for research.[2-5]

The National League of Nursing Accreditation Board is examining the research component of graduate programs in its institutional review process, reinforcing the acceptance of research as a major thrust of university nursing education. Similarly, the League and other professional groups, especially the American Association of Colleges of Nursing and the American Nurses' Association Commission on Nursing Education and Commission on Nursing Research, are concerned with the growth and development of doctoral programs in nursing—their mission, structure, financing, location, and output. The concern with nursing manpower nationwide, and especially at the advanced levels, spans 30 years. Dating from World War II and the immediate postwar era into the 1950s, surveys of nursing resources and studies of nursing activities were undertaken. Part of the impetus for these investigations came from experiences gained in administering the Cadet Nurse Corps program during World War II. The need for extensive research in problems of nursing practice and nursing education led to the establishment in 1955 of a program of nursing research grants in the Public Health Service. This was coincidental with a program of special fellowships for those nurses undertaking graduate preparation in research. In 1962, the research training capability went beyond support for individual nurses to include grants to institutions of higher learning, in support of research-related training in basic disciplines in or important to nursing. These institutional grants were called Nurse Scientist Graduate Training Grants, and provided not only for environmental support related to training activities, but also for support of selected numbers of nurse students in each grantee setting. Twelve universities and 260 trainees have received such federal support for research training, representing a total of $8,000,000 in expenditures for the period 1962 through 1976. Special Nurse Research Fellowships have provided support to 589 nurses for doctoral study for varying periods of time; these fellowships represent a total federal expenditure of $7,700,000 for the period 1955 through 1976.

A follow-up study of nurse fellows and nurse scientist trainees indicates that the majority of former fellows and trainees are engaged in teaching and research in academic settings, with the remainder conducting research or administering research programs in government and health care institutions. Universities remain the settings most earnestly in need of nurses with research preparation, but service settings are increasingly requesting nurses with doctoral preparation to head up research programs in patient care. Increasing demands for nurse doctorates was one of the topics discussed at a June 1974 Division-of-Nursing-sponsored conference on doctoral manpower requirements. It appears that the value of research and of research training for nursing is becoming recognized and endorsed. Federal support peaked in 1973 with 159 Fellows and 109 Nurse Scientists earning their doctorates. Since June of 1976, over 2,000 inquiries have been acknowledged from prospective research fellows and 120 new fellows are in various stages of study in the first quarter of 1978. As the input and the output from the research training programs has grown, staffs have witnessed a proportionate increase in the number and quality of studies dealing with aspects of nursing practice.

THE GROWTH OF PRACTICE RESEARCH

As recently as 1968, the lack of practice-related research was repeatedly addressed in the research literature, which included an overview of nursing research grants supported during the period 1955 through 1968; this overview was reported in a series of three articles published in 1970 in *Nursing Research*.[6-8] During the year 1970, the scientific review group charged with the review of nursing research grant applications took stock of the proposals before them, observing a wealth of problems suitable for study in the patient care arena and a serious dearth of appropriate methodologies and designs for problem resolution. A number of suggestions were forwarded for consideration by the Division of Nursing and by potential investigators. Among these were the establishment of research clinics, regionally and nationally, for criticism of research proposals, and increased consultation and assistance to potential investigators interested in practice-related research, both by governmental staff and by experienced investigators in academic and service settings. With increasing numbers of nurses receiving formal preparation in the techniques of basic biomedical and behavioral sciences, the period 1972–1976 showed a two-fold increase in the number of research grants dealing with clinical investigations directly related to aspects of nursing practice. The designs of this present group of clinical therapy studies are invariably experimental, indicating that we have overcome some but not necessarily all of the methodological problems that limited our earlier attempts to address aspects of nursing practice.

Because the scope of practice-related research has increased so dramatically in the last decade, an attempt was made recently to categorize such research into four major areas: (1) the science of practice, (2) the artistry of practice, (3) the structures needed for optimal delivery of patient care, and (4) the tools or methods needed for assessment of practice.[9] The definitions of each of these four areas, together with a definition of research utilization, are as follows.

Building a Science of Practice.   Studies that have as their primary focus the building of a science of practice through systematic identification of various characteristics, health problems, and health needs of patients and potential patients (individuals and groups), as well as aspects of relationships between nurses and patients, form a major category. Included in this category are studies concerned with differences in health needs and health problems among individuals in different groups; for instance, those of certain cultural and ethnic backgrounds, socioeconomic levels, age groups, and illness categories. Findings from these types of studies will enable us to better understand health care providers and the health problems and health behavior of the people.

Artistry of Practice. Another category has as its major thrust the refining of what we call the artistry of practice or clinical therapeutics, somewhat after Feinstein's usage of this term in medical care.[10] These are the laboratory and field studies that attempt to evaluate nursing procedures, techniques, and methods. Implied is a focus on what nurses do. These studies are of two types: (1) technical or physical procedures and (2) verbal, cognitive, psychosocial, and interpersonal aspects of nursing care. These two types are not fundamentally different; each deals with clearly specified nursing interventions and evaluates them in terms of patient outcomes. They differ only in type of intervention.

We would place in this group those studies aimed at reducing complications of hospitalization and surgical procedures as well as studies designed to evaluate different services or treatment primarily in terms of outcome. Additional studies are those designed to improve the outlook for high-risk groups such as the aged, the chronically ill, infants and mothers, and certain categories of families. There is an obvious relation among the group of studies that deals with science of practice, those studies that are directed toward refining the art of practice, and studies which are attempting to evaluate certain outcomes of practice as the dependent variables. Almost without exception the clinical therapy or artistry studies make use of an experimental design either in the laboratory setting or in the field, linking process and outcome. In group (1) are nursing technical procedures such as tube feedings, endotracheal tube care, tracheostomy care and suctioning, the administration of oxygen, and care of indwelling catheters. In group (2) are nursing interpersonal procedures such as teaching and counseling, which also address a process-outcome relationship.

Establishing Structures for Optimal Delivery of Care. A third category of patient care research is concerned with descriptive, analytical, and experimental studies of the physical and social environments in which nurses and their clients interact, as well as studies in which different patterns of health care providers are evaluated. Of particular interest are the structures that relate to service costs and relative efficiency.

Developing Methodology. A fourth category contains studies that aim to develop methodology or measurement tools, such as indicators of pain, quality of care, or knowledge.

Applications of Research Findings. Finally, there is another category of research that has potential for contributing to the improvement of patient care. It is a category in which we have virtually no current activities, but which might include studies that deal directly with the application of research findings to the field, through examination of such factors as single replications of an original design as well as wide-scale demonstrations. These studies often result in user manuals showing the practitioner how to study nursing activities in a patient unit or in an outpatient department or how to measure patient progress.

Model and theory development in nursing has assumed an increasing amount of attention. The Nurse Scientist Graduate Training Grant universities stimulated discussions about the science of nursing and the development of general theories of nursing through their annual seminars. These discussions culminated in 1969 and 1970 in a series of conferences on theory development held at the University of Kansas with federal support.[11] A review of the conference proceedings and of subsequent articles in *Nursing Research* suggests that there is still a good deal of debate about the desirable sources of nursing theory and the means for its development. There seems to be growing consensus, however, that the field of practice must figure prominently as the empirical source of many theoretical models and as the setting for their subsequent verification.

The author's preference regarding fruitful sources of nursing theory is sympathetic to the point of view taken by Ada Jacox in her recent article on this subject.[12] Her own work on pain is an excellent illustration of the potential contribution of nursing research to middle-level theories dealing with such clinically important problems as pain, suffering, and anxiety, in which the phenomena under study are investigated in such a way that the data allow for inferences and for inductive reasoning, thus leading to a growing body of scientific information. Thus the general category of model and theory development is diminishing as a separate category for our grant-supported work. Few studies have theory as their sole and exclusive thrust. The more usual occurrence over the past few years is that the clinical and laboratory studies directed towards aspects of nursing practice invariably have as a major purpose contributions to a science of practice and to theory development. In retrospect, the considerable interest in model and theory development in the late 1960s and early 1970s appears to have served a very useful purpose in highlighting the need to address this particular aspect in all research investigations. The scientific discourse between and among scientists also is growing so that a good deal of knowledge building is occurring that has not yet reached the printed page.

Regarding the artistry of practice, we have moved beyond exclusive reliance on descriptive research, which was felt to be the most direct line of attack to this particular problem in 1968.[13] Instead a variety of methodological approaches—experimental, descriptive, and historical—are being used in the development of nursing science. In addition, important theoretical models now available in the basic disciplines should be examined for their possible relevance to aspects of nursing practice, administration, and education. The fit won't always be perfect, but then the ultimate test of all theories will occur in their continuous refinement and applicability to fields of reality; in this instance, to nursing.

STRUCTURES FOR OPTIMAL CARE DELIVERY

With regard to the research category of structures for optimal care delivery, the last decade has been characterized by the development of several models for the delivery of a variety of services: urban and rural neighborhood health clinics; community mental health centers; out-reach programs and health care extension centers established by health professional schools and several major medical centers. Common to all these demonstrations is the provision of comprehensive health care for a segment of the American public at reasonable cost. Within this major mission, however, are several purposive subsets focusing around productivity, cost, quality, and target groups for whom special services are needed. Examples of these last are the aged, the chronically ill, infants and children, and families for whom the availability of supportive nursing services may be of greater importance than the availability of traditional medical services. Nursing research has examined the impact of nursing units such as the Loeb Center for Nursing at Montefiore Hospital in New York, the New Haven Hospice for the terminally ill, which developed from an interdisciplinary health care team, and nursing clinics primarily designed to afford health maintenance and primary care to the elderly. Progress has been slower in the acute care settings, yet there are projects underway to examine alternative structures for acute care management that will allow (a) improved quality of care and patient satisfaction for certain types of patients and (b) cooperative decision making and accountability among the health professions responsible for the provision of care. These were among the factors that led to the earlier success of specialized acute care units such as those for coronary patients and for the thermally injured. They are now among the factors associated with primary nursing.

It is important for nursing to recognize that it alone cannot resolve the problems associated with ineffective and inefficient health care delivery modes; it is but one of several provider groups and one that characteristically is lodged within highly structured or bureaucratic settings. To nursing's credit, however, is the fact that it encouraged and supported investigations into its services long before the field of health services research came into existence. In addition, several of the early studies by nurse investigators, behavioral scientists, and operations researchers contributed to the foundation of health services research through problem identification and methodological techniques.

RESEARCH ON QUALITY

Quality as a major focus of research into nursing care has been particularly noticeable in the past five years. Within this short period of time, a research conference brought together a small number of investigators to discuss the methodological problems in the field. The American Nurses' Association, the Joint Commission on the Accreditation of Hospitals, and the Division of Nursing, USPHS held national meetings to provide a forum for issues in quality assessment and assurance for health and nursing care. The Social Security Act amendments of 1973 established peer review organizations to monitor the need, use, and costs of services rendered Medicare and Medicaid beneficiaries, and several federally funded projects were launched to develop approaches to measuring the process and outcomes of nursing care. Among these last have been (1) the Rush-Medicus project that made the nursing process for inpatient care into a set of measurable criteria for use by hospitals; (2) the Wisconsin Regional Medical Program project to develop sets of patient health outcome criteria by nurse experts; and (3) the American Nurses' Association Health Services Administration contract to develop screening criteria and guidelines for peer review at the local level. There are individual publications of each of the above projects that the reader may find of interest.[14-17]

Particularly helpful as a summary of the issues is a recent monograph published by the American Nurses' Association, which contains the papers presented in December 1975 at an invitational conference on quality research.[18] The conference opened with a major paper by Avedis Donabedian and closed with remarks by Maria Phaneuf. Donabedian has proposed the following as particularly useful to all health fields in the area of quality assessment:

1. Further development of a measure of health status that could represent the final achievement of the health care system;

2. The devising of a battery of proximate, condition-specific outcomes that could be used to monitor and review the conduct of care;
3. Basic research into the process of clinical decision making so that it can be understood, and ways found to decide what are better ways of achieving specified goals;
4. Research that would result in better understanding of the professional-client relationship and attaching values to specified attributes of it;
5. Understanding the relationship between cost and quality, at the individual and aggregate levels, so that resource allocation decisions can be made rationally.[19]

The importance of participation by nurse researchers in quality assurance efforts is addressed by Maria Phaneuf in her concluding remarks. Of interest is the following:

> It seems sensible to suggest that some nurse researchers might concentrate on structure (S), some on process (P), and some on outcomes (O). The SPO approach is obviously applicable to the care of individuals, groups of individuals, in given settings, for total populations and for programs. This would mean that each group of researchers would deal primarily and clearly, though not exclusively, with the chosen component. The components are interdependent and interrelated, and for other obvious reasons, the three groups should work closely together toward the goal of synthesis and the development of quality assurance systems in which each component is subject to appropriate quality assurance methods of appraisal and evaluation.[20]

Consumer involvement in quality assurance efforts, accommodation of nursing specialization, development of a conceptual framework for peer review and explication of the core of professionals ethics or values remain problem areas in quality assurance, according to Phaneuf. To these the author would add several more, arising from the trial of the Rush-Medicus methodology in a professional standards review organization.[21] In that effort, which was the third phase of the quality monitoring study referred to earlier, a conceptual base for peer review in nursing was developed. It may serve as one model for professional review, along with others such as Lang's. The Rush-Medicus project also revealed that the issue is not really whether one approaches quality assurance research from the point of view of process or outcomes, or from a combined process-outcome approach such as suggested by Bloch[22] and Bellinger.[23] Rather it is to determine, for certain types of diagnoses or patient conditions or health states, what approach will be more valid or reliable than the other.[24]

Progress along this line has been hastened by increasing interest in developing taxonomies for nursing practice, such as nursing diagnoses, and by the use of standardized records, such as the problem-oriented record (POR). The last has been useful in the settings that have employed the POR as an aid in assessing patient progress and in facilitating interprofessional communication. The research on use of the nursing diagnosis is now in process; the development of classification schemes is a recent occurrence, and has largely been carried out with private resources through the efforts of a dedicated and concerned group of nurse investigators.[25]

Development of data bases, taxonomies, and techniques for measuring the nursing process and for assessing care outcomes are relatively recent trends, all occurring within the past few years, as nursing has become more assertive and articulate with regard to its special mission as a major health profession. It is important to note that these serve as research resources as well as means for greater professional autonomy and responsibility. Without these resources, and the persons skilled in their use, it would be difficult if not impossible to determine the nature and level of competence in nursing practice, to ascribe some social worth to this body of skills, and to make projections about manpower and training requirements.

PRIMARY CARE RESEARCH

Primary patient care has become the watchword of the seventies, and not surprisingly, research has been directed towards its implementation, its evaluation, and the mix of health professionals needed for its provision. A few significant studies in the 1960s signaled the advent of nursing's subsequent nurse practitioner movement. The Ford and Silver evaluation of post-training activities of pediatric nurses skilled in history taking and physical assessment revealed that they could handle independently three-fourths of clinic visits in one rural station and that patient satisfaction was high, particularly with regard to counseling and health monitoring.[26] These findings were confirmed in an adult ambulatory care center by Lewis and Resnik,[27] and again in another setting by Cheyovich, Lewis, and Gortner.[28] The Burlington randomized trials in Ontario carefully documented the impact on practice productivity, quality, and cost of the addition of family nurse practitioners to two solo office practices.[29]

As the issues of patient satisfaction and provider competence were resolved in these studies, the research questions have changed. Perhaps the most important current research question is the type or types of practice settings that will allow full opportunities for professionals to render a high level of care in accord with their training. The structural characteristics of ambulatory clinics, nurse-physician primary care teams, and health maintenance organizations that have gained recognition for effectiveness are being described in the literature, the most recent compilation being the Casebook of the National Joint Practice Commission.[30] Lewis[31] and Williams[32] commented upon the need for research on the influence of structural variables on nurse practitioner performance, noting methodological problems such as access to settings, overuse of research subjects and costs.

A second major research question in primary care deals with the problem of direct and third-party reimbursement for nurse clinicians and nurse practitioners. The Social Security Administration presently has underway a study of this issue for physician assistants and nurse practitioners.

A third major research question addresses the types of personal and professional characteristics that combine to make for effective and successful performance as a nurse practitioner. White has summarized well the state of the art in this area, and has called for research into the theoretical bases for adult personality change, for description of trait clusters that correlate with effectiveness, and from these descriptions the development of multi-criteria for measuring success and effectiveness.[33]

A fourth research question addresses the nature of the clinical judgments used by nurse practitioners and physicians working collaboratively in patient care management to (a) initially assign patients to a nurse or physician for primary responsibility, (b) reassign primary and secondary responsibilities as changes in patient progress or health states occur, and (c) develop their own management plans. The last involves the still elusive nature of the nurse-patient encounter—the process of care—from the initial plan, examination, questioning, and setting of priorities, to continued treatment, evaluation, and reappraisal. Few studies have been able to capture this process from encounter data or from patient records; perhaps it cannot be captured or quantified, for it does epitomize, in the best sense, the clinician-artisan at his or her work.

Finally, it has not yet been possible to develop a universal classification scheme of patient conditions, diagnoses, or problems suitable for nurse practitioner primary care management. This aim had been one of the original goals of the Cheyovich, Lewis, and Gortner study cited earlier. Although close to 800 patients' (veterans) records were surveyed independently by the nurse and physician to determine suitability for nurse practitioner management, conditions chosen represented multiple problems of a chronic, recurrent type such as hypertension, heart disease, arthritis, and diabetes, together with social and behavioral problems such as depression or anxiety. The difficulty encountered in determining the rationale for clinical judgments has already been cited as an area in need of research. It may be desirable to study the general range of problems and conditions most suitable for nurse practitioner management in those settings in which physicians and nurses are already in joint practice. In addition, for patients with multiple chronic conditions it is difficult to generalize beyond this single case, which has been the traditional clinical approach in both medicine and nursing.[34]

COMPETENCE

A research trend of increasing national interest is the appraisal of professional competence. Not surprisingly, research activities quickened with the need to establish the capabilities for sound clinical performance of nurses who were assuming such traditional medical skills as physical assessment and differential diagnosis. But impetus has come from other sources as well: (1) the movement in higher education toward competence-based learning and examination; (2) the development of non-traditional programs such as external degree programs; and (3) the concern for continuing education of professionals to assure safe and effective practice. It has been recognized for some time that the state board test pool licensing examinations measure cognitive knowledge and the understanding considered basic to safe nursing practice. The application of that knowledge and those understandings has been assessed infrequently in a systematic way, the most recent and interesting example being the clinical portion of the New York Regents external degree examination for associate degree graduates.[35] Several of the well-established nurse practitioner programs currently use simulated patient situations to assess clinical judgment, both in the form of paper and pencil tests and through actual subjects (who are normal volunteers). Others use actual patient situations and have the examinee do a complete workup. Interestingly, the author was tested by this last method twenty years ago upon completing the generic Master of Nursing program at what was then Western Reserve University.

As efforts move forward to develop better methods for evaluation of the professional performance of students, activities are underway to examine the performance of clinicians in practice. Perhaps one of the better known current efforts to appraise nurse practitioner performance is the project at the University of North Carolina dealing with family practice competence—the work here is basic enough to contribute to the field of family practice in general. Data were obtained from a national panel of physicians (generalists as well as specialists) regarding preferred treatment modalities for two indicator conditions, upper respiratory illness in children and the first year of life.

Treatment is defined as both treatment of the medical problem and treatment of the care needs. Additional activities are underway to assess decision making in the management of hypertension and to assess nurse-patient interaction in chronic diseases.[36]

Computerized programs of medical management for certain conditions or types of patients have been used by nurses to test their knowledge in these areas, often in connection with assignment to specialty units; one example recently given the author was the programs for coronary care management at Massachusetts General, now taken by house staff as they rotate through the service in order to identify teaching needs. Normative performance on these programs was provided by experienced coronary care nurses. The manually completed analog of these programs, including more nursing content, has been published as programmed instruction units in the *American Journal of Nursing* in recent years.

Finally, operational definitions of effective and successful nursing performance provided by a representative sample of generic nursing programs in the country were examined in a national study of prediction of successful nursing performance.[37] Criteria used by the schools to assess student performance, and to predict outcomes upon graduation, were compared with the self-appraisals of a cohort of their graduates six months into their first jobs, and with the appraisals of employers. The list of professional nursing activities developed to tap graduate performance may result in a worthwhile tool upon further evaluation. The response rate from employers of new graduates was remarkable (roughly a 75 percent return), suggesting that the topic of competence in practice is an important issue.

NURSING'S HERITAGE AND ETHICS

In recent years there has been a noticeable increase in the literature of articles based on the contributions of nurses during critical periods in the nation's history, of some of the early and prestigious schools of nursing, and of individual leaders in the profession who are credited with both the vision and activities that help to mold the development of nursing in this country. Concomitantly, there has been an increase in articles dealing with nursing's ethos, its philosophies for practice, and its theoretical propositions. Both sets of writings suggest that the sets of historical circumstances and the associated value systems that account for nursing's present state of affairs are being examined, not only to better document the state of affairs but also to identify those factors or variables that were or might be significant for continuing growth and development.

The investigator pool is small in both areas. Nursing history has but a handful of serious researchers at work: Teresa Christy, Philip and Beatrice Kalisch, Louise Fitzpatrick, and Gwendolyn Safier. Some of the problems associated with further development of the field are addressed in a recent publication by the Kalisches.[38] The methods of historical research are time-consuming, painstaking, and not easily delegated to research assistants. Hence a major problem lies in the inability of nurse historians and nurse historiographers to be freed from their regular academic or professional posts for sufficient periods to carry out a major scope of work. Very few professional schools currently offer courses in the history or philosophy of nursing (as was true 20 years ago), making it virtually impossible for faculty to combine their teaching and research activities. Research activities in nursing have a direct relationship to the importance ascribed to research by the professional leaders and practitioners. It is hoped that practitioners will recognize the potential harm being done to our professional heritage by the current lack of emphasis on both history and ethics, and take steps to redress the imbalance through support of research, teaching, and publication in these areas.

The area of values and philosophy has fared a little better as nursing has grown introspective regarding its special mission or ethos. Recent years have seen the publication of works by nursing's grand theorists—Rogers, King, Orem, and Roy—and some open forums on the development of nursing theories. The field of ethics and bioethics is virtually without activity or researchers, except for a small group of investigators and science administrators who have been concerned with and have published on the matter of human subjects in research. There are signs of heightened activity in this area, which are heartening, and which relate to public interest in the entire area of bioethics. The National Research Service Awards Act of 1974[39] established a presidential commission to study the issues concerned with the participation of human subjects in biomedical and behavioral research, including such controversial areas as fetal research, research on children, prisoners, and the mentally infirm, and psychosurgery. The commission has met monthly in open forums over the past several years to conduct its business, and the deliberations of this distinguished panel of ethicists, lawyers, scientists, and clinicians probably represent one of the most thoughtful and authoritative sources of information in the entire field of bioethics. There should be more opportunities provided for nurse scientists to have special training in these issues, in order to probe them more deeply through study and research. To provide stimulus for such study, the Division of Nursing, USPHS has listed bioethics as one of its major fields of predoctoral and postdoctoral research fellowships under the National Research Service Awards program, and became the first federal participating program to do so.[40] But again, the same constraints as noted for the development of historical research obtain: there is virtually no formal teaching of nursing ethics or philosophy (as distinct academic offerings) in schools of nursing, or for that matter in the other health professional schools. Not surprisingly there is virtually no research activity on the part of clinical scientists, whether these be nurses, physicians, dentists, or others working on health-related research, on major topics such as informed consent. The work done to date has been largely contributed by ethicists, and fortunately there are a few settings, such as the Kennedy Institute at Georgetown University and the Hastings on Hudson Institute in New York, that are sites of activity and that do provide for scholars in residence. If it is not yet possible for other settings to develop similar resources for bioethics, then perhaps interprofessional cooperation can be accelerated in the major health science centers to allow for the scheduling of interdisciplinary seminars, faculty contacts, and studies. It is the author's understanding that this type of activity is already underway in some settings; for example, the University of California at San Francisco. Through participation over the past years in the seminars on bioethics sponsored by the National Institutes of Health and the Kennedy Institute, through frequent observation at the meetings of the National Commission for the Protection of Human Subjects in Biomedical and Behavioral Research, and through limited contribution to the literature,[41,42] the need for far greater attention to ethics in practice and research has become apparent.

THE DEVELOPMENT OF RESEARCH RESOURCES

Perhaps the most significant and most auspicious trend in recent years has been the growth in resources for nursing research. These are varied but essential: the development of a small but critical mass of well-trained nurse investigators, increased communication within this group and productivity in terms of papers and publications, the emergence of professional and regional societies specifically concerned with nursing research, the growth of private and public funding sources for research, and the growth in the number of academic and clinical settings in which research activity is underway.

The size of the investigator pool is primarily a function of the size of the nurse doctorate pool, and this has grown steadily over the past decade and particularly in the past five years to bring the total number of doctorates to an estimated 1,800. Perhaps a third to a half of this number may be considered the active group of scholars, including investigators. The majority are lodged in academic settings as faculty, but an increasing number are in positions of research in service settings including large teaching hospitals, departments of public health, etc. Through their presence and activities they are creating favorable climates for research as well as directing their own research and advising others. The reinstatement of authority for support of research training for nurses at the predoctoral and postdoctoral level, through amendments to the National Research Service Award Act of 1974 (Public Law 93-348), will allow replenishment and extensions of the scientific talent needed for conduct of nursing research.

Communication among investigators, both formal and informal, is increasing through such means as scientific meetings and publications as well as correspondence. The Council of Nurse Researchers of the American Nurses' Association is the membership body of nurse researchers, and was established by the Board of Directors of the American Nurses' Association in 1970. The Commission on Nursing Research of the Association is the organizational successor to the earlier American Nurses' Association Committee of Research and Studies, and was authorized in the structure approved by the House of Delegates in the Bylaws. The Commission is the official policy voice for nursing research for the profession, and in its short lifespan has developed a number of important position papers in research priorities and preparation for research, as previously noted. The Council's annual program meetings address topics of interest to researchers, such as use of human subjects, and the membership can serve as a resource to the Commission.

The Western Society for Research in Nursing was formed under the sponsorship of the Western Interstate Commission for Higher Education's Nursing Council, which had been the sponsor for several years of federally supported research conferences. When federal support ended in 1974, the Society was formed to continue the efforts of communication and has held annual meetings since then which have been well attended. In the past two years, several Middle Atlantic schools of nursing have cooperated to hold annual research conferences for investigators located in the East. In addition to these efforts, several university schools hold special research conferences on particular topics, and their local Sigma Theta Tau chapters have sponsored the conduct of research days such as those held each year at New York University. Finally, and perhaps most important, research papers have begun to be presented at the conventions of the American Nurses' Association and the National League for Nursing, and both organizations have gone on record as endorsing research as an essential part of professional education and practice.

Support for institutional research activities began with the creation of the Institute for Research and Service in Nursing Education at Teacher's College, Columbia University, and was soon followed by the establishment of the department of nursing within the Walter Reed Army Institute of Research. Although both of these units were the source of important studies, Werley has noted the circumstances that hindered the growth and expansion of these activities: too few nurse investigators prepared to handle complex clinical problems; too few resources available to make use of potentially rich clinical settings; and too narrow a perspective on the part of those involved to make use of opportunities.[43]

In order to overcome some of these limitations, the federal government began a program of environmental support in 1958 to upgrade faculty skills in nursing research and to provide needed resources such as consultants, supplies, and equipment. Between 1958 and 1966, 21 awards were made with the following outcomes noted: recruitment and retention of research-trained faculty; time and opportunity to participate in exploratory studies, some of which dealt with aspects of patient care; the availability of consultation in the form of a qualified project director; the availability of supporting services; stimulation of ideas and creation of a favorable research climate; and establishment of a timetable or program for research. Since 1966 the program of environmental support has increasingly emphasized actual conduct of research, and in recent years the participation of service settings has increased.[44]

Finally, the growth of financial resources for nursing research has increased over the years, and these resources have become better known to potential grantees. Increasingly, nurse scientists are making use of university intramural funds as well as extramural funds such as federal research grants and private grants. In Fiscal Years 1977 and 1978 the federal authorization specifically earmarked for nursing research stood at an all-time high of $5,000,000 for research grants and $1,000,000 for research fellowships, a tribute to the efforts of those whose work and activities in the fields of nursing research and resource development in research have gained national recognition.

AN HISTORICAL PERSPECTIVE

The emergence of nursing research within the past few decades as a field of inquiry pursued by nurse scientists and by other investigators interested in health and illness care was preceded by a half century of professional growth. In a recent documentation of the history of research in nursing in this country,[45] note was taken of the fact that early studies were undertaken to resolve problems seen as major concerns of the times: the control of communicable diseases in the first two decades of the century (with emphasis on hygiene, sanitation, proper asepsis in the home, where the bulk of surgical procedures was still carried out, and maternal and child health); documentation of appropriate nursing procedures and case management for difficult patient care situations; the transfer of nursing services from the home into the hospital; the development of appropriate curricula for the education of students and graduates; and the improvement of the social and economic welfare of the profession.

These last two concerns were seen as mutually interdependent, i.e., improvement in the profession would follow improvement in education for the profession. Accordingly, a number of national surveys were sponsored to obtain needed data.

The first national survey of schools of nursing in the United States was undertaken for the Federal Bureau of Education by Adelaide Nutting in 1912. The responses of 1,100 participating schools revealed nursing education to be predominantly utilitarian and undistinguished with regard to its quality. The next national survey was financed by the Rockefeller Foundation in 1923 and included a sample of schools of nursing as well as private duty nurses and public health practitioners. The recommendations from this study, now known as the Goldmark Report, were impressive in urging shortening and enriching of the basic curricula, in advocating the growth of university-based programs that would combine general education with professional education, and in noting that some nursing tasks could be delegated to attendants. To address the quality of nursing education, a national committee on the grading of nursing schools was established by the National League for Nursing in 1926, and a director was named (May Burgess) to undertake studies that would: (1) establish supply and demand for nursing services; (2) conduct job analyses of nursing and nurse teaching; and (3) conduct an actual grading of nursing schools. All were accomplished with the exception of the actual grading, although schools were advised of the weaknesses noted in their programs in comparison to other schools. These included inadequate educational resources, too heavy an emphasis on hospital work, and too little emphasis on public health or home care. Following the completion of these studies, the League undertook publication of three standard curriculum guides, the last of which represented a major research effort.

Hence these early studies were prompted by concerns of the early nursing leaders and professional organizations about the quality of nursing education and nursing practice, and about the economic status of the profession. The national surveys were directed by non-nurses and financed by philanthropic groups. This pattern continued into the midcentury, and resulted in additional fact-finding studies, one of the most notable being Esther Lucile Brown's *Nursing for the Future*.[46] The shortage of professional nurses had become acute during the World War II period, and insufficient supply was to become one of nursing's most persistent problems. The Ginzberg report,[47] published the same year as the Brown report, recommended that the shortage be eased by the development of technical nursing programs of two years' duration, with professional programs extended to four years. Interest in the placement of technical nursing programs in community colleges was stimulated by this report.

Six national nursing organizations formed a joint board of directors to implement the Brown report, and the board was eventually named the Committee for Improvement of Nursing Services. Inherent in this title was the assumption strongly held by the nursing leaders for the greater part of this century that improvement of nursing education would lead directly to improvement of nursing practice, and that the last was dependent on the first. The Committee undertook a survey of all state-approved schools of nursing, and developed an initial classification of the schools according to predetermined criteria. A followup was intended and undertaken by the National Nursing Accreditation Service, with assistance from private foundations. The Service was taken over by the National League for Nursing in 1952, and since that time a voluntary program of accreditation has been available for baccalaureate and higher degree programs, for diploma programs, and for associate degree programs. Presently there is interest in researching the validity of accreditation criteria.

During the 1950s studies continued in order to develop functions, standards, and qualifications for practice for each of the major nursing interest and specialty groups. These studies were sponsored by the national nursing organizations, and this period came to be known as the activities studies period. Also during this time the first known attempt was made to establish minimal requirements for nursing services in hospitals.

Marking the culmination of several decades of effort to improve the structure and quality of nursing education, the early 1960s became known as the peak period for studies of student characteristics, including student recruitment and retention and prediction of student performance. In addition, initial attempts to study nursing's process of professional socialization were undertaken. While interest in educational research remains, the focus has shifted somewhat in recent years to address the criteria of effective practice, as associated with the performance of practitioners rather than students.

In 1961 a prestigious interdisciplinary group was established to advise the Surgeon General of the Public Health Service on nursing needs and resources, and on the appropriate role of the federal government in assuring adequate nursing services in the nation. The Surgeon General's Consultant Group strongly supported nursing research and the training of nurses in research methods, and it recommended increased funding levels for extramural research grants and research fellowships, as well as the availability of consultation and institutional assistance. Finally, it was recommended that a national study be undertaken "of the present system of nursing education in relation to the responsibilities and skill levels required for high quality "care."[48] Both national nursing organizations joined forces to establish a commission for the Study of Nursing and Nursing Education that would serve as an independent agency to carry out the study, with a named director (Jerome F. Lysaught), and to secure funds (made available by the Kellogg and Avalon foundations and a private individual). During the period 1967 through 1970, the study was carried out and subsequently published as *An Abstract For Action.*[49] The commission found that changes in nursing practice and nursing education would need to follow three major thrusts: (1) increased research into both the practice of nursing and the education of nurses; (2) enhanced educational systems and curricula based on results of that research; and (3) increased financial support for nurses and nursing to insure adequate career opportunities. An implementation phase was undertaken following the completion of the major study in 1970, in order to (1) develop and expand nursing practice, with particular attention paid to relationships among the health professions; (2) repattern educational systems to meet current needs and to allow innovation; and (3) further the development of a strong profession ready to fully accept its mandate for service and accountability.

In 1975, a contract was negotiated between the Western Interstate Commission for Higher Education and the Division of Nursing, Department of Health, Education, and Welfare to plan, analyze, and project distribution of nursing personnel skills and services on a nationwide basis; develop analytic tools for planning at state and local levels; conduct pilot tests; develop data bases; carry out needed demonstrations of improved services; and develop training programs and centers for nursing leaders.[50] The study has been concluded and the final report is being readied for publication. Two national conferences were held in 1975 and 1976 to acquaint nurse planners, policy makers, nurse educators, nurse service providers, state legislators, and representatives from state and local agencies with activities and findings from the project. State models for planning have been developed, as has a national model, together with an Inventory of Innovations and Demonstrations in nursing care delivery. Most problematic to date have been the data bases, because of local, state, and regional variations in collecting and maintaining statistics on nurse supply and distribution. For example, there has been a time lag of over four years since the last published inventory of nurses with earned doctorates. It is therefore difficult to draw a cohort of nurse Ph.D.s who earned their doctorates between the years 1972 and 1975 for follow-up survey by the National Academy of Sciences Committee on a Study of the Nation's Needs for Biomedical and Behavioral Science Personnel. National concerns over governmental invasions into the public's privacy through surveys, use of identifiable data such as social security numbers, and maintenance of computerized lists and records has made difficult the conduct of government-initiated and -sponsored data collection surveys. As policy decisions rest increasingly on data to support particular positions (e.g., the relative efficacy of home care for the renal dialysis patient; third party reimbursement of health professionals [other than physicians] who are now primary care providers; the procedure of choice for decubitus ulcer management; alternatives to institutional care for the aged; etc.) the need for careful research continues. And without a diminution of the basic research that has led, often serendipitously, to medical and scientific advances, increasing attention must be directed to the clinical sciences and the nursing and health services research areas to provide the knowledge from which sensible judgments can be made. The final quarter of the twentieth century may well see nursing as a major contributor to research in health care. The time is ripe and the work is long overdue.

REFERENCES

1. S.R. Gortner, "Research for a Practice Profession", *Nurs Res* 24 (May–June 1975): 193–97.
2. American Nurses' Association Commission on Nursing Research, *Nursing Research, Towards a Science of Health Care* (Kansas City, Mo.: American Nurses' Association, 1976).
3. ——, *Priorities for Research in Nursing* (Kansas City, Mo.: American Nurses' Association, 1976).
4. ——, *Preparation of Nurses for Participation in Research* (Kansas City, Mo.: American Nurses' Association, 1976).
5. ——, *Human Rights Guidelines for Nurses in Clinical and Other Research* (Kansas City, Mo.: American Nurses' Association, 1975).
6. F.G. Abdellah, "Overview of Nursing Research 1955–1968," Part I, *Nurs Res* 19 (January–February 1970): 6–17.
7. *Ibid.,* Part II, *Nurs Res* 19 (March–April 1970): 151–62.
8. *Ibid.,* Part III, *Nurs Res* 19 (May–June 1970): 239–52.
9. S. Gortner, D. Bloch, and T. Phillips, "Contributions of Nursing Research to Patient Care," *J Nurs Adm* (March–April 1976): 22–28.
10. A.R. Feinstein, "What Kind of Basic Science for Clinical Medicine?" *N Engl J. Med* 283 (October 1970): 847–52.
11. C.M. Norris (ed.), *Nursing Theory Conference, 1st, 2nd, and 3rd Proceedings,* held at the University of Kansas Medical Center Department of Nursing Education, March 20–21, 1969; October 9–10, 1969; and January 29–30, 1970 (Kansas City, Kansas: the University of Kansas, 1970).
12. A. Jacox, "Theory Construction in Nursing: an Overview," *Nurs Res* 23 (January–February 1974): 4–13.
13. F.G. Abdellah, "Overview of Nursing Research 1955–1968," Part I, *Nurs Res* 19 (January–February 1970): 10.
14. R.C. Jelinek, R.K.D. Haussmann, S.T. Hegyvary, and J. Newman, *A Methodology for Monitoring Quality of Nursing Care.* HEW Publication No. (HRA) 74-25, Washington, D.C.: USGPO, 1974.
15. R.K.D. Haussmann, S.T. Hegyvary, and J. Newman, *Monitoring Quality of Nursing Care, Part II: Assessment and Correlates.* HEW Publication No. (HRA) 76-7, Washington, D.C.: USGPO, 1976.
16. M.J. Zimmer, N.M. Lang, and D.I. Miller, *Development of Sets of Patient Health Outcome Criteria by Panels of Nurse Experts,* Final Report of

Project #7 (Madison, Wisc.: Wisconsin Regional Medical Program, 1974).

17. American Nurses' Association, *Guidelines for Review of Nursing Care at the Local Level*, Washington, D.C.: USGPO August, 1977.

18. American Nurses' Association, *Issues in Evaluation Research*. An Invitational Conference, December 10–12, 1975. (Kansas City, Mo.: American Nurses' Association, 1976).

19. A. Donabedian, "Some Basic Issues in Evaluating the Quality of Health Care," in *Issues in Evaluation Research*. An Invitational Conference, December 10–12, 1975. (Kansas City, Mo.: the American Nurses' Association, 1976), p. 25.

20. M. Phaneuf, "A Concluding Paper," in *Issues in Evaluation Research*. An Invitational Conference, December 10–12, 1975. (Kansas City, Mo.: the American Nurses' Association, 1976), p. 141.

21. R.K.D. Haussmann and S.T. Hegyvary, *Monitoring Quality of Nursing Care, Part III: Professional Review for Nursing: An Empirical Investigation*. HEW Publication No. (HRA) 77-70, Washington, D.C.: USGPO, 1977.

22. D. Bloch, "Evaluation of Nursing Care in Terms of Process and Outcome: Issues in Research and Quality Assurance," *Nurs Res* 24 (August 1975): 256–63.

23. A. Bellinger, "An Examination of Some Issues Pertinent to Evaluation Research and the Assessment of Health Care Quality," in *Issues in Evaluation Research*. An Invitational Conference, December 10–12, 1975. (Kansas City, Mo.: the American Nurses' Association, 1976), pp. 115–27.

24. S.R. Gortner, "The Quest for Quality." Invitational paper for the 1976 American Nurses' Association Convention Program, sponsored by the Commission on Nursing Research, Atlantic City, New Jersey, June 1976.

25. K. Gebbie and M.A. Lavin, "Classifying Nursing Diagnosis," *Am J Nurs* 74 (February 1974): 250–53.

26. H.K. Silver, L.C. Ford, and L.R. Day, "The Pediatric Nurse Practitioner Program: Expanding the Role of the Nurse to Provide Increased Health Care for Children." *JAMA* 204 (April 27, 1968): 298–302.

27. C.E. Lewis, B.A. Resnik, "Nurse Clinics and Progressive Ambulatory Patient Care," *N Engl J Med* 277 (December 7, 1967): 1236–41.

28. T.K. Cheyovich, C.E. Lewis, and S.R. Gortner, *The Nurse Practitioner in an Adult Outpatient Clinic*. HEW Publication No. (HRA) 76-29, Washington, D.C.: USGPO, 1976.

29. W.O. Spitzer et al., "The Burlington Randomized Trial of the Nurse Practitioner," *N Engl J Med* 290 (January 1974): 251–56.

30. The Casebook project is under compilation. Address inquiries to the National Joint Practice Commission, John Hancock Center, Suite 1864, 875 North Michigan Avenue, Chicago, Illinois 60611.

31. J. Lewis, "The Structural Aspects of the Delivery Setting and Nurse Practitioner Performance," *Proceedings of the Nurse Practitioner Research Conference I* (University of Connecticut Health Center, Hartford, 1974).

32. C.A Williams, "Nurse Practitioner Research; Some Neglected Issues," *Nurs Outlook* 23 (March 1975): 172–77.
33. M. White, "The Personal and Psychological Characteristics of Applicants to and Graduates of Nurse Practitioner Programs," in L. Hochheiser et al: *Proceedings of the Nurse Practitioner Research Conference I* (University of Connecticut Health Center, Hartford, 1974).
34. T.K. Cheyovich, C.E. Lewis, and S.R. Gortner, *The Nurse Practitioner in an Adult Outpatient Clinic,* HEW Publication No. (HRA) 76-29, Washington, D.C.: USGPO, 1976.
35. C.B. Lenburg, "The External Degree in Nursing: the Promise Fulfilled," *Nurs Outlook* 24 (July 1976): 422–30.
36. E.H. Wagner et al, "Influence of Training and Experience on Selecting Criteria to Evaluate Medical Care," *N Engl J Med* 294 (April 15, 1976): 871–76.
37. P. Schwirian, *Prediction of Successful Nursing Performance,* Parts I and II. HEW Publication No. (HRA) 77-27, Washington, D.C.: USGPO, 1977.
38. B. Kalisch and P. Kalisch, "Is History of Nursing Alive and Well?" *Nurs Outlook* 24 (June 1976): 362–69.
39. Public Law 93-348, "The National Research Service Awards Act of 1974."
40. Bureau of Health Manpower, Division of Nursing, *National Research Service Awards for Individual Predoctoral and Postdoctoral Nurse Fellowships,* HEW Publication No. (HRA) 76-76, Bethesda: USGPO, 1976.
41. S.R. Gortner, "Death with Dignity: Ethical Issues in the Proposed Legislation," in *American Nurses' Association Clinical Sessions* (New York: Appleton, 1975).
42. S.R. Gortner and D. Bloch, "Ethical Aspects of Nursing Practice," videotape unit in the series *Nursing and the Law* (New York: American Journal of Nursing Company, Education Services Division, 1974).
43. H. Werley, "This I Believe About Clinical Nursing Research." *Nurs Outlook* 21 (November 1972):718–22.
44. S.R. Gortner, "Research in Nursing, the Federal Interest and Grant Program," *Am J. Nurs* 73 (June 1973): 1052–55.
45. S.R. Gortner and H. Nahm, "An Overview of Nursing Research in the United States" *Nurs Res* 26 (January–February 1977): 10–29.
46. E.L. Brown, *Nursing for the Future* (New York: Russell Sage, 1948).
47. E. Ginzberg, *A Program for the Nursing Profession* (New York: MacMillan, 1948).
48. Surgeon General's Consultant Group on Nursing, *Toward Quality in Nursing: Needs and Goals.* Washington, D.C.: HEW, 1963.
49. The National Commission for the Study of Nursing and Nursing Education, *An Abstract for Action* (New York: McGraw-Hill, 1971).
50. "Analysis and Planning for Improved Distribution of Nursing Personnel and Services," National Conference, Western Interstate Commission for Higher Education, Boulder, Colorado, November 1976.

CHAPTER TWO

EDUCATIONAL ISSUES RELATED TO RESEARCH IN NURSING

Virginia S. Cleland

During the 1980s, graduate faculties in nursing will develop many new doctoral programs, several of which will be Ph.D. programs aimed at preparing nurses for research and teaching positions as graduate faculty members in universities. The education of advanced practitioners, educators, administrators, planners, and evaluators must be considered along with that of researchers. However, the development of science underlying the practice of nursing is so fundamental to the work of all nurses that it can be appropriately given special attention in this book.

In the first section, attention will be directed to graduate education programs for the total profession. Succeeding sections will focus upon educational preparation for nursing researchers.

PROGRAMS AND DEGREES

Probably nothing can be written about academic degrees which a reader cannot compare to an example that contradicts. Such societies as the Council of Graduate Schools in the United States (CGS) and the Association of Graduate Schools in the Association of American Universities have made recommendations about degree structures,[1,2] but the universities can do as they think best. In some instances, patterns currently at variance with CGS recommendations were established by prestigious schools before any policy was enunciated. In other cases, political power struggles on a local campus have produced decisions which override rational judgement. In still other situations logic can justify either of two alternative positions.

The Doctor of Philosophy (Ph.D.) degree is recognized as the highest academic achievement for creative original scholarship and research. While some academicians have maintained that it should be awarded only for basic research, this position is not supported by the arbiters of such disputes: "The Doctor of Philosophy shall be open as a research degree in all fields of learning, pure and applied."[1]

Nursing should attempt to keep its degree structures within the policy positions of the CGS. The Ph.D. degree program is approved by a university's graduate council. Professional degree programs can generally be initiated following approval by a school's faculty. A program which should lead to a Ph.D. degree by reason of the research competencies expected should not award a professional degree simply to avoid having to obtain program approval from a university's graduate council. Because it is misleading, it is inappropriate for a professional school faculty to state they have a research program if, in fact, the graduate council of that university will not so label the program.

Stephen Spurr's book, *Academic Degree Structures*,[3] makes clear the important distinctions between the professional doctorates which reflect preparation for entry into the profession—e.g., the Doctor of Medicine (M.D.), Doctor of Dental Surgery (D.D.S.), and Juris Doctor (J.D.)—and professional doctorates which reflect advanced specialized preparation for persons who have entered the profession at an earlier or lower academic level—e.g., Doctor of Public Health (D.P.H.), Doctor of Business Administration (D.B.A.), and Doctor of Education (Ed.D). The professions have found that it is not possible to prepare for occupational entry and leadership in a single degree program. Medicine has met its need for advanced practitioners through professional specialty certification rather than through advanced degrees. Some medical and law schools award master's degrees for advanced study, acknowledging that the professional doctorate reflects entry level preparation rather than graduate education.

The National Association of Social Workers agreed in 1970 to admit to full membership individuals who obtained a bachelor's degree in an undergraduate program of social welfare, as well as those with traditional master's level preparation.[4] This change occurred when the Association could not prevent the hiring into social welfare positions of workers without the M.S.W. degree. The Association had united behind a high standard of professional education but could not meet the societal demand with workers prepared at that level.

The change was also supported because the profession had no academic setting in which to prepare teachers, administrators, and practice specialists. The Ph.D. was an inappropriate degree for producing the numbers of social workers needed for leadership positions within that profession.

Schools of public health have for decades admitted students from the health professions with earned baccalaureate, master's, or doctoral degrees and who have begun studies in public health in M.P.H. programs with the option of continuing to the D.P.H. for high level leadership positions. The Ph.D. degree has been retained as the research degree.

From its roots in philosophy, psychology evolved into a natural science with a strong academic tradition. World War II fostered the development of *clinical* psychology because, in the military services and in the Veterans Administration hospitals, psychologists were permitted to practice psychotherapy in addition to administering and interpreting personality and intelligence tests. With the enormous growth of clinical psychology, the discipline of psychology found it had given birth to a profession. In 1976 there were five professional schools of psychology. These schools are not awarding the traditional Ph.D. degree because their faculties believe the dissertation requirements for that degree are irrelevant. Instead they are awarding the Doctor of Psychology as a more appropriate degree for professional practice.[5]

These examples are cited to illustrate that each profession, within the framework of higher education, has adjusted its graduate programs to meet the societal demand for its services. The profession retains its authority as long as society supports its methods as effective and efficient. Society finds ways to circumvent the profession's policies if these are irrelevant or insensitive to social demand.

There are two distinct doctoral degrees which have been utilized in nursing: the Doctor of Nursing Science (D.N.S.), which is a professional degree, and the Doctor of Philosophy in Nursing (Ph.D.), which is an academic degree. The professional doctoral degree is granted by the nursing school. These programs, founded in the 1960s, were generally established for one or more of the following reasons: (a) there were inadequate numbers of Ph.D.-prepared people in the nursing faculty and inadequate programs of faculty research for university graduate councils to approve a Ph.D. program; (b) nursing school faculties sought to establish school-controlled programs rather than those controlled by universities to avoid irrelevant language requirements and similar problems; and/or (c) the faculties wanted to prepare nurses for advanced leadership positions other than that of researcher and wished to avoid unreasonable standards for dissertation research.

Simultaneously, with the initiation of D.N.S. programs, there developed, under the federal support of the Nurse Scientist Graduate Training Grant, programs in which qualified graduate students in nursing were financially supported in a Ph.D. program in a discipline related to nursing. The Nurse Scientist programs and the Special Nurse Research Fellowship programs (both supported by the Division of Nursing, HEW) produced a cadre of nurses who, while earning their Ph.D. degrees, became well trained in the research process.[6] The influence of these nurses as members of graduate faculties has greatly altered graduate education in nursing. Now, in the 1970s, several university nursing schools have established or are planning to develop doctoral programs which will award the Ph.D. degree.

While the Ph.D. degree is the recognized degree for the preparation of researchers, is it the only advanced graduate degree needed by the profession? The need for nurses prepared for leadership positions with advanced graduate degrees will be so great, if the Ph.D. degree is the only option, that the demand will go unmet. Unfilled positions will be absorbed by such other professionals as hospital administrators and allied health educators. One alternative is to lower the standards of the Ph.D. degree in nursing and grant the degree for completion of courses and examinations rather than for the development of research competence. Use of this alternative would, however, seriously impede the further development of nursing research.

It is inappropriate to equate preparation for advanced leadership positions with research preparation. For the profession as a whole, as in a faculty organization, it is the total mix of available competencies which is important. All nursing faculty members should be scholars but not all need to be researchers. The profession needs scholarly researchers, scholarly practitioners, and scholarly adminsitrators. The profession needs nurse researchers in order to develop areas of nursing knowledge, but it would be a grave mistake to believe that every practitioner, administrator, or educator needs to be a researcher. The profession does not now and may never have the resources to develop, in all of the nurses needed for professional leadership, the sophisticated research competencies which the Ph.D. degree should reflect.

The D.N.S. degree is a very appropriate advanced degree. Professional doctorate programs are usually of shorter duration than the Ph.D. program administered by professional schools, and in time they will be submitted for accreditation by appropriate professional bodies. The curricula are developed to meet the profession's needs for advanced practitioners, administrators, health planners, and evaluators and are built upon the sophisticated practitioner's programs evolving at the M.S.N. level. The degree recipients can be expected to be knowledgeable in the theory and processes of nursing practice and in the theory and processes of the functional area of choice. The D.N.S. degree reflects specialized graduate study and as such can open the door to many employment options. Because it is built upon a baccalaureate nursing degree, it has wide recruitment possibilities.

Rozella Schlotfeldt has proposed that the optimal preparation be a baccalaureate degree (B.S. or B.A.) before entry into professional nursing.[7] She suggests that a few schools adapt their programs to the needs of such students and grant a Doctor of Nursing (D.N.) degree. For such students the D.N. degree would be the first professional degree in nursing and would be awarded concurrently with license to practice. This, Dr. Schlotfeldt believes, is the appropriate route if nurses are to be prepared for entry into scholarly practice the same as members of other learned professions. The graduates of such a program would, like physicians and lawyers, have to seek graduate specialty education in other master's and doctoral programs. These programs would be somewhat like the early Yale University and Western Reserve University programs for college graduates. At present no school is awarding a D.N. degree.

The professional doctorates (D.N. and D.N.S.) and the academic doctorate (Ph.D.) each reflect programs which can meet professional needs.[8,9] If each is available, the integrity of the others is protected. Nursing need not restrict its offerings but it is important that each program be certain of its particular goals and be stalwart in its mission when recruiting students.

As indicated earlier, this first section of the chapter has been to describe the nature of graduate programs and advanced degrees needed by the profession for its human resources. The remainder of the chapter will pertain only to Ph.D. programs and to preparation for research in nursing.

FACULTY RESOURCES

The abilities of the faculty form the single most important resource in the development of a graduate research training program (Ph.D.). A faculty lacking in either quantity or quality should lead schools to exercise caution in making a commitment to a doctoral program. Such decisions would be easier to make if all graduate faculty members possessed doctoral degrees and if all persons who had earned a doctorate had also developed research competence, but neither proposition is true.

One issue faced by a faculty is whether all faculty members possessing earned doctorates can be viewed as resources for a doctoral program.[10] The answer is clearly "No." The assessment of competence can be made, in part, by examining the research and scholarly productivity of faculty members. To begin a small program, there should be at least four to six faculty members who have had postdoctoral research experience and who can direct dissertation research. There should be another eight to ten doctorally prepared faculty members without such well-developed research skills, but possessing other capabilities needed in a graduate program in nursing.

Unless there is considerable ongoing research within the faculty, it is unlikely that a suitable environment for research training can be produced. The Division of Nursing, HEW initiated the Faculty Research Development Grants in 1958 and replaced this with the Research Development Grants in 1966 for the purpose of developing research activity within faculty organizations.[7] The effect of these grants in developing the research capability of one faculty has been well described by Rozella Schlotfeldt in *Creating a Climate for Nursing Research.*[11]

Because no school has the research depth it would like, the profession needs to develop cooperative mechanisms for sharing research talent. There are several models already in existence which could be utilized in interschool cooperation.[12-14] Other examples are:

The Cooperative Graduate Education in Nursing (COGEN) project of California and Nevada, formed in 1971 as an interinstitutional consortium involving 12 universities. Cooperative activities are extensive and have included the development of teaching modules for nursing research, faculty exchange, and student exchange.[15]

The Michigan Intercollegiate Graduate Studies (MIGS) program, a cooperative arrangement among the public-supported universities in Michigan. MIGS enables a student on one campus to register for selected graduate courses on another campus. When the course requirements have been completed the course credit appears on the home school transcript. This permits registration for courses not available on the home campus or for one being taught by a "noted" faculty member on another campus.[16]

The "Big Ten" graduate schools of the Midwest, Committee on Institutional Cooperation (CIC). Through CIC, mechanisms exist for student and faculty exchange. Nursing schools in the Midwest with graduate programs have been exploring the relevance of these mechanisms for doctoral education for nurses.[17]

Each university has its own structures which can support or retard institutionl cooperation. The procedural problems usually can be solved if sharing is desired. In order to have the broadest possible selection of appropriate nurse researchers for a student's dissertation committee, methods for sharing should be explored. Many qualified researchers are underutilized as teachers because there is no doctoral program on their particular campus, or students in a faculty member's area of expertise.

Another issue related to the use of faculty resources pertains to the number of doctoral students at the dissertation level whom a faculty member should advise. In a paper given before the Council of Baccalaureate and Higher

Degree Programs of the National League for Nursing (NLN) in Houston in 1976, this writer stated:

> Within colleges of nursing, the senior faculty members who will be involved with doctoral programs tend to carry very heavy service responsibilities in the profession, in the college, and in the university. While we as faculty are learning what is involved in preparing good clinical researchers, let us hope no faculty member will direct more than two dissertations simultaneously. Later, if a faculty member finds that the nature of his or her workload or the nature of the knowledge area or the type of research methodology permits advisements of more students, allow the ratio to rise to 1:5 or so.[10]

Faculties may tend to make too sharp a distinction between courses in the master's program versus those in the doctoral program. It is probably better to consider the courses as graduate rather than as belonging exclusively to one program level or another. A doctoral student may need clinical courses which are taught by master's-prepared faculty members. Students who have graduated from one-year master's programs are likely to need greater clinical depth, as will be true of the student who wishes to change or broaden the area of clinical specialization.

In time, all graduate faculty members in nursing will possess a doctorate, but to hold to that rule today would remove many excellent faculty members who through extensive study have developed sophisticated theoretical knowledge in their clinical areas. These persons must not be replaced until there are applicants with doctorates who have comparable clinical competence. Further, the scarce faculty resources for doctoral programs must not be dissipated by service on excessive numbers of professional, university, and college committees. Dr. Kalisch, in her article, "Creativity and Nursing Research," has written convincingly:

> In our tendency to overorganize everything, there is great excess of committee work, meetings, communications, and schedules that eat away at our time and with which we complicate our existence. Other distractions, including crushing teaching or service loads along with outside activities such as consultation and workshops, usually force the nurse to bog down at the very threshold of the research arena.[18]

STUDENTS

There are no substitutes for intelligence and motivation in doctoral study and research. The problem is to identify these characteristics with some validity. Past performance is generally the best predictor of future performance, but grade inflation, prevalent since the late 1960s, has obscured the value of honor point average (HPA) as a criterion. It is a fairly common practice to require an HPA above 3.0 at the undergraduate level and 3.5 (4.0 = A) in previous graduate studies with some exceptions made on the strength of other attributes in the record.

Tests such as the Graduate Record Examination (GRE) or the Miller's Analogies Test are generally required as part of graduate admission to provide the admissions committee with information about applicants' general aptitudes. The Division of Nursing, HEW, probably has collected the most data on GRE test scores for nursing doctoral applicants. These data have not been made public, but Dr. Bourgeois has reported, "The majority of fellowship applicants hold total scores ranging from 1,000 to 1,350."[19] A student with quantitative scores between 450 and 500 and with higher scores in the verbal area may need a slower-paced research sequence than a student who received higher quantitative scores. This seems to be a reasonable alternative for students who show high potential in all other areas. It is not unusual for applicants with quantitative scores below 450 to have more of an orientation towards practice than towards research. Sometimes this may be the clue that the nurse should be applying to a program leading to a professional degree.

The personal interview and written goal statement are valuable for assessing research interest and motivation. Some applicants state quite frankly that they are unwilling or unable to tolerate much stress and ambiguity on the way toward the degree. Applicants who must set such limits probably should not be admitted to research programs, since unpredictability is the only predictable matter in scientific investigation.

The influence of previous work experience on doctoral study has not been assessed. Because research questions tend to grow out of past experience relived with new theoretical insights, clinical experience would seem highly desirable. Applicants who have done considerable teaching or have been involved in educational administration tend to want to ask educational questions which are inappropriate if the program goal is to produce clinical or patient care research.

An important issue relating to doctoral study pertains to the place of full-time versus part-time study. Base level financial support is available through National Research Service (NRS) awards for individual predoctoral and post-doctoral nurse fellowships.[18] The Nurse Training Act of 1975 makes Title II

Traineeships available for award by approved graduate nursing programs. Both award mechanisms, administered by the Division of Nursing, can be extended for a total of 36 months of graduate study. The NRS awards are particularly useful for nurses seeking degrees in sciences related to nursing or in health services.

Therefore at this writing (1976) monies are available. However, the nurse may not want to give up a current position, or may have made financial commitments to a higher standard of living, or may not wish to ask the sacrifice of her family that a full-time program requires. As long as financial support is available and faculty resources are in such short supply, it would seem professionally undesirable for graduate programs to admit part-time students. To provide maximum interaction between faculty and students, there should be many hours of mutual availability.

Because nursing has been blessed with considerable federal support, graduate assistantships in teaching and in research have not been developed by graduate programs in nursing. The two types of assistantships most often derive from quite different financial sources.

The graduate assistantship in research usually is made available through funded research projects where the graduate student can obtain valuable "on-the-job" training, working with a senior investigator. Worthen and Roaden, who studied research assistantships, concluded:

> Research apprenticeship experience offered in a university is apparently related positively to the number of graduates entering research careers (when systematic research training was incorporated as part of the assistantship). In addition, persons who hold genuine research assistantships are found after graduation to spend more time in research, complete and produce more research studies, and produce studies of above average quality. If these are—as we believe them to be—desired outcomes for programs designed to produce researchers, then the research assistantship would be an integral part of every such program. Of course, this assumes intelligent tailoring of research assistantships to offer the types of valuable experiences* . . . The mere existence of employment and financial aid opportunities labeled "research assistantship" has little training value.[20]

The graduate assistantship in teaching derives from institutional "teaching monies." A faculty instructorship may be divided into two graduate assistant-

---

*The research assistantship must provide supervised research training and not be just a source of financial support.

ships in teaching. The student engages in the teaching role for half time and carries a reduced study program. In many disciplines the graduate assistantship has been an unsupervised teaching experience designed to reduce faculty teaching loads and provide support for graduate students.

Graduate programs in nursing could provide teaching assistantships of considerable value to students who have never taught or who have never taught in a university setting where the faculty role in its entirety can be observed or experienced. Such assistantships may meet the need of mature students who need more income than a fellowship can provide. If properly structured and supervised, a graduate assistantship in teaching can provide considerable socialization into the role of an academician.

Perhaps students who receive federal traineeships or fellowships without any employment obligation should have 8 to 12 hours per week of supervised research training included in their program of study. Nurse faculty members fully appreciate the need for field practice in the development of clinical skills, but have not provided students with the equivalent opportunities to develop research skills. The dissertation experience is very valuable, but it is not enough. Field practice in research must be incorporated into the nursing Ph.D. programs for students who do not receive the experience of working as a graduate assistant in research. The socialization of graduate students into the role of a research investigator is a significant part of research training.

CURRICULUM

Within nursing there has been no professional agreement on the nature of the program of study in preparation for nursing research. However, if one were to examine the graduate level transcripts of nurses who are making or have made a contribution to the development of nursing research, one would find a common base of preparation. There are differences in labeling and there are differences in scope and depth, but differences in the nature of the content are not great. Each nurse's graduate studies would include learning experience in the nature of knowledge, research methodology, nursing, and a related discipline.

Although at present there is great ambiguity, there is also great opportunity to put units of learning together in imaginative ways. There are no professional edicts which say certain contents should be included. The standards for graduate education as developed by the American Nurses' Association's Commission on Nursing Education can be met in many different ways.[21]

The broad general areas of course content are described below. It should be noted that these descriptions refer to a student's total graduate program;

i.e., master's and doctoral. The content may have been included one place or another, but somewhere at some time a researcher in nursing needs preparation in these areas. It is also assumed that the nurse would possess a B.S.N. degree, or its equivalent, obtained in the undergraduate program in an NLN-accredited school of nursing.

Nature of Knowledge. One portion of the graduate program should include preparation in philosophy of science, theory development, conceptual frameworks, and the nature of knowledge and its organization. This type of content is often taught in departments of philosophy, but is probably better taught with nursing as the central focus because of the abstract nature of its content. While this material will appear in many courses, it is important that doctoral students obtain in-depth experience in this area.

Research Methodology. Another component of the curriculum is composed of research methods, design, and statistics which enable the student to design and conduct systematic inquiry. A doctoral student should have completed a minimum of two or three courses beyond the first course in inferential statistics which, today, is probably included in all M.S.N. programs. Analysis of variance is valuable for its contribution to the understanding of research design as well as statistical analysis, per se. Non-parametric statistics are important to include because of the wide usage of these techniques in clinical research, where the investigator is often forced to work with small samples. Advanced work in research methods and design can be incorporated into doctoral seminars pertaining to theory and research in a particular content area.

Nursing Science. Nursing is probably the most difficult area for the faculty to conceptualize as a coherent whole. Faculties who do this generally ignore the realities of a medically controlled health care system. The fact remains that patient admission, placement, treatment, and discharge are medically controlled. To ignore these facts is to live in academic isolation.

If the nursing program is organized without regard for medical specialties as they exist in health service institutions, it becomes difficult to prepare nurses for specialty practice. Society has developed a long history of circumventing groups not responsive to its needs. The majority of M.S.N. programs are first organized in the pattern of the "medical model," and then use a conceptual framework for nursing within that clinical area.

The organization of nursing at the master's level into areas of practice makes it difficult to organize nursing at the doctoral level into areas of knowledge appropriate as a focus for research. Practice areas invariably include several areas of knowledge, for practice can rarely be so limited and specialized. Death and dying form a knowledge area which would be applicable in many practice areas.

At Wayne State University, the faculty is developing two- to four-credit seminars to delve deeply into theory and research in particular areas. The knowledge areas derive from faculty interest and research and, unlike a curriculum, have no other unifying framework than practice relevance. There is no reason to believe that faculty research will develop or should develop within one particular conceptual framework. However, each faculty researcher will have a personal conceptual framework for nursing practice which directs the search for researchable problems. Theory selection or development will most often derive from that conceptual framework. Participation in two or three such seminars is expected to provide the doctoral student with sufficient background to pursue a related path of inquiry, or to develop a similar base in another problem area.

Related Discipline. Nursing science is an applied science which derives in part from the underlying basic sciences upon which practice is built. Nursing, like dentistry, medicine, education, or engineering, draws assumptions and utilizes concepts, constructs, and propositions from other fields of knowledge. Each profession develops its own practice science.

In most doctoral programs the student is required to take some course work in an outside department, in a field of knowledge related to his own discipline. This serves at least two purposes: (a) to broaden the base of knowledge (theory and research methods) and (b) to enable the student to view the development and organization of knowledge in another area (process).

For these same reasons, doctoral students in nursing profit in having a related discipline included with the program of study. Nurse scientist programs were developed by including the entire doctoral program of the related discipline. This was done at great sacrifice of time and energy directed toward the development of nursing science. A reasonable alternative is the incorporation of a substantial minor consisting of those courses in the related discipline which contain the theory and research which the nurse doctoral student wishes to utilize in an area of research. Depending upon the student's background in the related discipline, there may be need for three to six courses to give the student the necessary facility to use that discipline in nursing research.

PROGRAM SUPPORT

It is important that Ph.D. programs in nursing are not established on grant money. A nursing faculty needs to know whether its university administration is willing to use its own money to fund the program, and whether the graduate council will approve the program without monies from outside the institution influencing the decision.

If the program can only be initiated on soft monies, it should not be started. A doctoral program requires a great commitment from the faculty members involved. Research programs are difficult to move to another campus. It is unfair to request this level of involvement if, in fact, the program could be terminated by the failure of a grant renewal.

A doctoral program which has a sufficient base of support from university monies to enable the faculty to admit four to six students per year is secure enough to seek outside funding to enlarge the program, and to add faculty members with special talents. If the outside funding is withdrawn the program may be cut back in size but it can continue. Also, the reader is referred again to the suggestions given in the prior section of this chapter pertaining to faculty. The sharing of scarce resources through collaborative efforts between universities must be encouraged. Society cannot afford for nursing to do otherwise.

Where faculty and financial resources are inadequate for a doctoral program in nursing, it would be better for the school of nursing to refer doctoral inquiries either to Ph.D. programs in disciplines related to nursing or to doctoral programs in nursing on other campuses. Underfinanced and understaffed programs will produce poor doctoral education which in turn leads to poor nursing research or, more frequently, the absence of nursing research. The profession needs large numbers of nurses with doctorates to fill the leadership positions. The numbers of active, productive nurse researchers will remain relatively small; they should be prepared with great care under optimal conditions.

REFERENCES

1. The Council of Graduate Schools in the United States, *Policy Statements Concerning the Nature and Naming of Graduate and Professional Degree Programs* (Washington, D.C.: The Council of Graduate Schools in the United States, 1969).
2. The Council of Graduate Schools in the United States, and the Association of Graduate Schools in the Association of American Universities, *The Doctor's Degree in Professional Fields* (Washington, D.C.: [Undated]).
3. S. Spurr, *Academic Degree Structures; Innovative Approaches and Principles of Reform in Degree Structures in the United States,* prepared for the Carnegie Commission on Higher Education (New York: McGraw-Hill, 1973).
4. A. Gurin and D. Williams, "Social Work Education," in E. Hughes (ed.),

Education for the Professions of Medicine, Law, Theology, and Social Work, prepared for the Carnegie Commission on Higher Education (New York: McGraw-Hill, 1973).

5. D. Peterson, "Is Psychology a Profession?" *Am Psychol* 31 (August 1976): 572–81.

6. E. Vreeland, "Nursing Research Programs of the Public Health Service," *Nurs Res* 13 (Spring 1964): 148–58.

7. R. Schlotfeldt, "Research in Nursing and Research Training for Nurses," *Nurs Res* 24 (May–June 1975): 177–83.

8. Bureau of Health Manpower Education, Division of Nursing, *Future Directions of Doctoral Education for Nurses.* Washington, D.C.: HEW, 1971.

9. J. Matarazzo and F. Abdellah, "Doctoral Education for Nurses in the United States," *Nurs Res* 20 (September–October 1971): 404–14.

10. V. Cleland, "Basic Considerations in the Development and Implementation of a Doctoral Program in Nursing," *Nurs Outlook* 24 (October 1976): 631–635.

11. R. Schlotfeldt, *Creating a Climate for Nursing Research* (Cleveland: Case Western Reserve University, 1973).

12. R. Frey, "Cooperation in Doctoral Programs Among Universities of the Committee on Institutional Cooperation," *Dissert. Abs. Int.* 34 (1974): 4781A.

13. R. Lancaster, "Interdependency and Conflict in a Consortium for Cooperation in Higher Education: Toward a Theory of Interorganizational Behavior," *Dissert. Abs. Int.* 31 (1970):619 A.

14. L. Patterson, "A Descriptive Study of the Governance of Selected Voluntary Academic Cooperative Arrangements in Higher Education," *Dissert. Abs. Int.* 32 (1972): 3628A.

15. S. Chater, "COGEN: Cooperative Graduate Education in Nursing," *Nurs Outlook* 23 (October 1975): 630–32.

16. ——, *Michigan Intercollegiate Graduate Studies (MIGS)* (Lansing: Michigan Council of State College Presidents, 1973).

17. H. Grace, *A Study of Resources for Doctoral Education in Midwest* (Evanston, Ill.: Committee on Institutional Cooperation, 1975).

18. B. Kalish, "Creativity and Nursing Research," *Nurs Outlook* 23 (May 1975): 314–19.

19. M. Bourgeois, "The Special Nurse Research Fellow," *Nurs Res* 24 (May–June 1975): 184–88.

20. B. Worthen and A. Roaden, *The Research Assistantship* (Bloomington, Ind.: Phi Delta Kappa, 1975).

21. Commission on Nursing Education, *Standards for Nursing Education* (Kansas City, Mo.: American Nurses' Association, 1975).

CHAPTER THREE

SUPPORT FOR AN EMERGING SOCIAL INSTITUTION

Joanne S. Stevenson

Earlier in the evolution of the Nursing Research Movement in the United States, emphasis was put on providing informational, educational, socio-emotional, and/or financial support to nurses who evidenced researcher-like potential. The major thrust of the research support efforts was focused at the individual level—that is, to promote the development of *individual* nurse researchers. Targeting research support and development efforts directly at this level should continue, but in a lower priority position than heretofore. Much more time and energy should be channeled into external system influence on behalf of nursing research by organized segments of the nursing profession.

It is not individual researchers per se who should be the focus of research support efforts for the next several years. Rather, nursing research, or more accurately a *social institution* called Nursing Research, is the more appropriate target for organized nursing's support efforts. Individual researchers and individual research projects could thus automatically be given the support they require within a total-system approach to development of such a social institution.

Certainly the goal of all the individual efforts and various phases of the nursing research movement since the early 1950s could be defined as the eventual institutionalization of nursing research. The ultimate hope has been to make nursing research a natural, expected, commonplace, and traditional basis for nursing. Success in this enterprise would mean that at some future time the term *nursing research* would not raise eyebrows, that it would become an unobtrusive concept, fade out of the realm of *extra*-ordinary experience and move into the realm of everyday vernacular. Research-based nursing practice would be the *traditional* mode and experiments would be conducted to test newer forms of research-based practice against *older* forms of research-based practice. Newer theories would be tested through research and accepted, revised, or discarded on the basis of how they fared under the rigors of the research process. Nursing faculty members in academe would be socialized into expecting themselves and their colleagues to be productive researchers. Remedial efforts to prepare nurse-faculty to learn how to become researchers through the mode of continuing education or inservice education would be passé. Research development efforts would be channeled into the training of students in research and the facilitation of the efforts of seasoned nurse researchers. Nursing has already covered a large percentage of the distance toward the goal of institutionalizing nursing research. The position taken here is that a great deal more effort along the paths taken so far will produce diminishing returns unless the policymakers, the funding agencies, and the public change their attitudes. Organized nursing can do this if it will reframe the basic plan and change the primary target from individual nurses to the non-nursing environment.

SYSTEM LEVELS

Institutionalization of nursing research is a goal that requires several identifiable multilevel support systems. One can dare envision and write about such an institution in the late 1970s because of the progress made in nursing research development since the early 1950s. Today many people in nursing accept without question the need for research-based practice.

Explicit evaluation of the progress of nursing research over the past 25 years shows different results depending on the biases of the evaluators. Despite slowness of growth, uneven quality, minimal quantity, questionable relevance, and disappointing lack of impact on nursing practice, it has evolved. One would be hard-put to deny that fact. The present status of nursing research is very different from its status in 1950. Hence the profession can set its sights differently now. While development of individual researchers and support of individual research projects must always be a priority, these should become ordinary expectations of nursing education, service organizations, and clinical practice. A broader focus really should be embraced by the nursing community as a whole. Development of nursing research as a national and an international social institution should replace the more individualistic person-level focus of earlier times.

The highest system level for research support activities to be addressed in this chapter will be the national level, in this instance the United States. Extrapolation of these comments to the international level would be an interesting undertaking but that is beyond the scope of this chapter.

Several identifiable organizations at the national level have been supportive to nursing research and should be encouraged to continue and expand their efforts at the larger-system level. Others have not been supportive but could be under a less restrictive interpretation of their stated mission.

The discussion of national level organizations begins with the American Nurses' Association and then goes on to the National League for Nursing, the American Association of Colleges of Nursing, Sigma Theta Tau, and several other formal or informal groups of nurses. Throughout this discussion funding agencies and foundations outside nursing are discussed vis-à-vis their track record of support to nursing research and the chances of enhancing their support in the future. A recommendation is made to nursing groups about enhancing their influence in the arena of extra-nursing research support systems.

After covering the major agencies at the national level, the discussion moves to nursing groups at the state and regional level. Regional organizations are discussed, followed by groups organized through the state nurses associations. Suggestions are made for consolidating the individual efforts of these many groups in order to increase the efficiency of their work and produce a collective impact.

Research support at the local level is presented by using the district nurses association as a prototype of local nursing organizations. The research support responsibilities and possible strategies of organizations and agencies which employ nurses are discussed at some length, including structural changes, centralized research subsystems, and normative re-educative, power coercive, and peer support strategies in the framework of planned change.

The chapter ends with a discussion of the individual level; that is, the potential or actual nurse-researcher level. Support and development strategies useful for helping both neophyte and seasoned researchers are presented. Individual nurses can, for example, exert influence on local agencies, foundations, or associations to view nursing research in a more favorable light. Some tactics for effecting such changes are listed and discussed.

National Level

American Nurses' Association. The primary responsibility for the institutionalization of nursing research into the profession of nursing rests unequivocally with the American Nurses' Association (ANA) as *the* professional organization and voice of organized nursing. The ANA's support of nursing research is a well-documented historical fact. Some of the most notable recent ANA contributions include: creation and financial backing of the American Nurses Foundation (1955); planning and direction of the federally funded ANA Research Conferences (1965-74); creation of the ANA Commission on Nursing Research (1970); creation of the ANA Council of Nurse Researchers (1972); encouragement of state nurses' associations to set up state and regional councils; and the creation of the American Academy of Nursing (1974). Paradoxically, creation of these research sub-systems can be viewed both positively and negatively. They are only sub-systems with specific goals and tasks to perform. The ANF, for example, is not guaranteed a share of ANA membership fees. It has actually never been clear that the ANA itself, as the collective conscience of professional nursing, behaves as if it was committed to scientific inquiry as the sine qua non of nursing practice. Indeed the contrary is true. Decisions made within the ANA sometimes support and sometimes hurt the institutionalization of nursing research.[1] Hence, those sub-systems of the ANA which were created to enhance nursing research are faced with a dual function like the Greek god Janus. They must look *inward* and try to aggrandize the importance attached to nursing research internally with the central leadership and the membership of the ANA. Simultaneously, they must look *outward* to the non-nurse support systems comprised of legislators, other professions, private research foundations, health-care agencies, and the consumer public. This type of two-headed effort is frustrating and time consuming; progress is painfully slow and backsliding is frequent. However, since nursing research is not yet an institutionalized expectation either within the nursing community or outside of it, both target populations must be educated and persuaded simultaneously.

ANA Commission on Nursing Research.   In May 1970 the ANA Commission on Nursing Research was created to formulate the ANA's policy on research, as well as its priorities for research, and to stimulate the conduct of nursing research. The Commission has in recent years put considerable time and energy into the development of a national legislative program to support research in nursing. Two specific strategies included publishing a booklet about nursing research for public relations use and developing a network of nurse-researchers for legislative action. It is not clear how much actual ANA clout goes with the commissioners in their meetings with congressional representatives. It is also not clear how much local constituency clout is attributed to each commissioner by the congressmen from their home territory. These two things are not separate. If the ANA had a more powerful image, and if ANA power was truly behind research in nursing, then influence on the legislators would be more substantial than it currently appears to be.

In addition to the executive and legislative branches of the federal government, the Commission could do more to influence two other research support systems in the United States in an attempt to open up these systems vis-à-vis monetary support for nursing research. One target would be the bureaucratic machinery of the Health component of the Department of Health, Education, and Welfare (HEW). Within the United States Public Health Service (USPHS), in particular, there are numerous institutes, branches, or divisions which are apathetic, oblivious, or openly negative toward nurse-initiated proposals. Individual nurse-investigators may occasionally be funded, but that does not eliminate the systematic exclusion of nursing research under their program priorities. It also does not change the tradition that only credentialed medical practitioners are acceptable principal investigators. Opening up the closed doors requires either so much power that others must pay attention or strategic use of small amounts of power. Either way, power does not belong to and cannot be energized by individual investigators; the expertise of professional lobbyists is needed for the planning and timing of such efforts and the clout of a big organization is required for any change to be effected.

Another set of research support organizations, which should be influenced by the ANA through the ANA Commission on Nursing Research, is composed of the national research foundations that support health- or illness-related research. Certainly private foundations have funded nursing in the past, but these grants were for studies of nurses as an occupational group, of the educational practices of nursing schools, or for scholarships to basic and graduate students. Most foundations have guidelines that exclude clinical nursing research either explicitly or implicitly. Explicit exclusion is easy to spot in their statement of purposes or statement of research interests. Implicit or de facto exclusion is more difficult to discern but it can be implied from long-term absence of support to any nursing study even though the written policies do not exclude nursing or nurses explicitly. A major effort should be made by organized nursing at the national, state, and local levels to gain access to the foundations and the voluntary agencies which sponsor health-related research at the parallel levels; i.e., the national, regional, state, and local levels. One very important goal would be to broaden foundation policies and practices so that nursing proposals would be welcomed and given a fair review. Another would be to loosen written or unwritten rules about credentials and disciplinary background of the principal investigator. Most foundations still act as if the only credential appropriate for a principal investigator is an M.D. Finally, the resources of the ANA should seek to reframe the focus of the foundations and voluntary associations from a narrow concentration on causes, cures, and symptom-control to a philosophy that would embrace research on health maintenance, disease prevention, and living with chronic conditions. It is amazing how many associations founded by persons with a particular condition focus their support on irradication and fail to support those who are living with that condition in the present.

Basically, the major sources of private research funding can be dichotomized into: (1) the family and corporate foundations which were created to manage the distribution of a portion of the family fortune or corporate profits. Their goals emanate from some interest area designated by the founder and interpreted by a Board of Trustees; and (2) the national headquarters of voluntary organizations created to alleviate one or more specific disease(s) or condition(s). Examples of private foundations and organizations that could profitably be approached include: the Robert Wood Johnson Foundation, the American Cancer Society, the American Heart Association, the Ford Foundation, the Rockefeller Foundation, the Millbank Memorial Fund, certain of the drug, medical supply, and hospital equipment companies' foundations.[2,3]

The ANA Council of Nurse Researchers. The ANA Council of Nurse Researchers represents a worthwhile attempt by the Commission on Nursing Research to provide a reference group, a forum and meeting ground, where strangers meet and collaborate around common interests. The major achievement in the first few years after 1971 was a sense of group identity for the nation's pool of active nurse-researchers. Primary reference groups are extremely important, especially in an environment of apathy, negative reinforcement, pejorative behavior, or outright punishment to nurse-researchers. A primary reference group can be a sustaining force, even if it only meets once or twice a year.

In addition to the reference group function, the Council meetings are forums for researchers to report on newly initiated, in process, or completed studies. It is a social atmosphere where doctoral students can rub shoulders with established researchers and get oriented to the national nursing research network. It is a place for persons with doctorates in basic sciences to become resocialized as nurse-researchers. In addition to the formal program of each meeting, the informal getherings and discussions which take place among participants are potent aides to self-identification as a constituent in a community of nurse-researchers. Socialization, affirmation, and identification of members as nurse-scholars by other members is crucially important to the continued viability of the small minority of nurse-researchers in this nation.

The Council engages in multiple activities and services which directly serve the Council members, including a newsletter with items of information to the membership. The Council and the Commission should develop more of a partnership to develop and implement strategies directed toward opening up more sources of research funds to nurse-researchers. The Commission's goal of developing a legislative network should be expanded to other forms of influence and to include private funding sources. The Council members could be its soldiers in this campaign.

The National League for Nursing. The National League for Nursing (NLN) has in the past contributed to the evolution of nursing research in a variety of ways. The League was instrumental in getting various foundations to sponsor early studies in nursing. It obtained a grant from the Commonwealth Fund in 1955 to support a fellowship program for nurses with aptitude for research careers. The NLN is credited with initiating the publication of *Nursing Research.* The League seemed to reverse itself about valuing nursing research during the period between 1965 and 1975. Even the criteria for accreditation of baccalaureate and higher degree programs in nursing did not contain the word research. Happily, the draft criteria which will be implemented by the League in 1978 do contain several references to research; as a support responsibility of administration, as a faculty activity, and as a student activity. The new NLN criteria come closer to giving such attention to scholarly activities as befits an academic unit in an institution of higher learning.

New Groups on the Scene. Two other groups of highly educated nurses which should be included in any discussion about support for nursing research are the American Association of Colleges of Nursing (AACN) and the Principal Investigator and Project Directors (PI and PD) group of the Research Development Programs in Nursing funded through the USPHS Division of Nursing. The AACN has been a politically active group since its inception. Annual meetings are held in Washington, D.C. and include group and individual discussions with lawmakers. The fifth objective in the articles of the Association is to influence governmental policy with respect to the advancement of education, research, and service in nursing and to improve health care for all people.

The AACN has become more politically astute through trial and error dealings with lawmakers and governmental personnel. To date, this group has not put much energy into support for nursing research; however, they indirectly lobby for nursing research through their efforts to improve the funding base for graduate programs, graduate student traineeships, and pre-doctoral fellowships to nurses. Hopefully, as more of the colleges become involved in doctoral education, this group will step up its efforts to get larger allocations into the federal budget for nursing research.

The PI and PD group is not an organization, but rather an informal aggregation of nursing research administrators and developers who meet once a year to help each other through sharing successful approaches to research development in their local areas. Over the past several years this group has become increasingly involved with tactics to increase the funding base for nursing research. Its members have also tried to increase the number of nurses in decision-making positions in HEW. They have tried to inform the Secretary of Health, Education, and Welfare about the availability of highly qualified nurses in ever-increasing numbers who could be appointed to peer review committees, advisory councils, consultant positions and ad hoc groups within HEW. They have also expressed concern about the trend toward more managers and fewer professionals in top-level HEW positions. So far the group has relied on letters to various organizations and individuals to convey its recommendations. The responses have not been encouraging.

NURSES SUPPORT THEMSELVES

The American Nurses Foundation. The American Nurses Foundation (ANF) was founded in 1955 by the American Nurses' Association as a way to organize a continuing, fulltime, coordinated program devoted to nursing research. The Foundation is supported through the contributions of individual nurses and of corporations, which include regular contributions from the ANA and the American Journal of Nursing Company. Other corporate contributors include a few drug companies, medical equipment companies, and the like. The foundation funded just under 100 projects between 1955 and June 1976 in patient care and health care research. Individual awards are limited to one year of $5,000, including indirect costs. Second-year renewals for an equal amount are possible, subject to competitive review of a second application. There is a need for such small grants in nursing but there is a definite limit to how much the profession can depend on such a small foundation to support its vast need for research monies.

The ANF has become more aggressive in recent years in soliciting contributions from corporations and national foundations. It should become a middleman between researchers and the big foundations. The ANF is another voice which could become more active in convincing large foundations and private philanthropists of the potential benefits of investing in health research and patient care research implemented by nurse investigators.

Sigma Theta Tau. Sigma Theta Tau is a national nursing honorary that was founded in 1922 at Indiana University. One of its purposes is to stimulate research in nursing and to this end it established a research fund in 1936. The first practice-oriented research project was funded in 1938; the second one was funded in 1966. Awards made between 1936 and February 1966 were for scholarships, educational research, or studies of nurses. The 1938 grant was to develop a teaching manual for diabetic patients. The 1966 grant went to Rita Chow for an investigation entitled: "Identifying Nursing Action With the Care of Postoperative Cardiac Patients."[4]

The total number of projects funded between 1936 and 1976 is approximately 90. Since 1966 the trend has been toward funding more clinical studies. The dollar amount per grant is small. Sigma Theta Tau is growing rapidly and the number of projects funded each year has been steadily increasing. There is, however, a finite limit to how much it can do to support nursing research in the broader sense, unless it takes a more active part in promoting nursing research to the public, to foundations, and to governmental bodies. Sigma Theta Tau directly and/or indirectly through its Research Fund Committee could become partners with the other representatives of nursing research interests in the United States.

FEDERAL GOVERNMENT AND NURSING RESEARCH

USPHS Division of Nursing.   The Division of Nursing within the United States Public Health Service, Health Resources Administration, Bureau of Health Manpower administers the Nursing Research Program for the federal government. Budgeting for research training and the conduct of research studies has been capricious over the years since 1960. The advantage to having the Nursing Research component in the Division of Nursing is that the Division maintains an identity with nursing and hence there is a strong tie to Nursing Research—the disadvantage is that research as an expected activity is not an integral part of the Bureau of Health Manpower. As a consequence, it is often difficult to make a case for a research budget as a line item and several times in recent years there has been *no* line budget item for nursing research in the budget of the Bureau of Health Manpower. If the research component of the Division of Nursing was transferred elsewhere, say to the National Institute for General Medical Sciences, the research funding base might be strengthened and clarified in the bureaucratic hierarchy. Even crumbs in the institutes can be significant amounts of money. However, the continued viability of nursing research as an identifiable disciplinary entity might be put in serious jeopardy in the institutes.

The federal interest in and commitment to nursing research deserves more assistance from the nursing community. Other professions and special interest groups have pushed hard in the past and continue to push hard to aggrandize federal programs which match their vested interests. It is foolhardy for nursing to expect federally employed nurses to be the prime movers in infuencing legislators toward more programs and larger allocations for nursing research and research training.

Several other components of the USPHS will accept and review protocols submitted by nurse-researchers. The National Center for Health Services Research (NCHSR) reviews a wide variety of proposals from all health disciplines. The basic mission of the Center is to sponsor research on the spectrum of issues directly related to some aspect of health service delivery. The priorities are: quality of care; inflation, productivity, and costs; health care and the disadvantaged; health manpower; health insurance; planning and regulation; ambulatory care and emergency medical services; and long-term care. The Center is, perhaps, too much of a catch-all and it has stringent standards about the multi-disciplinary mix required to do health services research. The Center has funded nurse principal investigators but would not fund a study that lacked a multi-disciplinary team approach.

Another potential avenue for support lies in the Division of Long-Term Care. This is a very new entity which existed as a part of the NCHSR until June 1976. The focus of this division is on delineating national problems, issues, and unmet needs concerning the delivery of long-term care services and the status of research, education, and technical assistance activities in the long-term care field. It will be receptive to investigations about long-term care regardless of the specific discipline of the principal investigator, but again, the emphasis is on multi-disciplinary research.

The National Institutes of Health (NIH) seem to be showing some signs of openness to nurse investigators. The Institute of General Medical Sciences, the Institute of Heart and Lung, and the National Cancer Institute appear to be increasing their interests in post-hospital maintenance, quality of life, and several epidemiological issues about causative factors. The National Cancer Institute's Cancer Control Program frequently distributes Requests for Proposals (RFP's) that could be of interest to nurse-researchers. One way to keep informed of the changing interests of the institutes is to get on the mailing list of the specific institute that best suits your interests. The *Commerce Business Daily* carries complete listings of all new federal interests and Requests for Proposals. Most universities subscribe through their central grants office. Nurse-researchers should direct persons in the grants office to alert them to any items in the *Commerce Business Daily* which contain certain key words that match their research interests.

Regional and State Levels

Regional Groups. Regional consolidation has been a long time goal of the Western Interstate Commission of Higher Education in Nursing (WICHEN). In the early years the focus was on nursing education but very early in the Nursing Research Movement WICHEN became a powerful promoter of nursing research in the western region which consists of these 13 states: Alaska, Arizona, California, Colorado, Hawaii, Idaho, Montana, Nevada, New Mexico, Oregon, Utah, Washington, and Wyoming.

WICHEN has been the recipient of many research grants and manages the formidable task of getting people from several states to produce at an unbelievable rate of speed during a two- or three-day face-to-face meeting. The WICHEN Research Conferences are a well entrenched tradition and recently their sponsorship has been taken over by the Western Society for Research in Nursing. It is difficult to project what will happen to the research division of WICHEN in the next several years without the core support of the Research Development Grant. It could survive and thrive if core support under a new program of institutional grants becomes available.

The Southern Regional Education Board (SREB) represents 14 states in the southeastern United States, including: Alabama, Arkansas, Florida, Georgia, Kentucky, Louisiana, Maryland, Mississippi, North Carolina, South Carolina, Tennessee, Texas, Virginia and West Virginia. The interst of SREB in nursing education is old, but their interest in research is new. In 1974, a survey of research activities in the South was completed and published under the title, "Nursing Research in the South, A Survey."[5] The SREB developed a regional plan for research development and obtained a grant from the USPHS Division of Nursing in February 1977 to implement this regional plan.

The Committee on Institutional Cooperation (CIC) is a consortium in the Midwest composed of the Big Ten universities (Illinois, Indiana, Iowa, Michigan, Michigan State, Minnesota, Northwestern, Ohio State, Purdue, and Wisconsin) and the University of Chicago. In 1973, meetings began between representatives from the graduate programs in nursing in the CIC about regional planning for doctoral programs. Since issues related to nursing research were so closely intertwined with doctoral program planning, the discussions included regional concerns about nursing research, preparation of researchers, research space, facilities, equipment, libraries, and supplies with particular emphasis on sharing resources and avoiding the pitfall of unnecessary and expensive duplications. This group is still in the very early stages of regional collaboration. The deans of the CIC schools, which also belong to the AACN, have been meeting about their mutual interests and concerns. There was also one meeting of the deans, the educators, and the PI and PD group from the CIC schools. These groups have not yet had time to develop a crystallized set of goals and strategies, but they have at least made a beginning.

State Councils. State nurses associations remained aloof from research development processes until very recently. At the ANA Convention in June 1974, a resolution was passed by the Council of Nurse Researchers that interest groups for nurse researchers be formed within the state nurses associations. The state of Michigan had already started development of a state council. Ohio and Illinois developed state level groups during the summer of 1974. Other states have followed through with the recommendation more slowly.

The state councils could function in ways parallel to their national counter-parts vis-à-vis statewide sources of research funding, state agencies, state departments of health, state legislators, the executive branch of state government, statewide private research foundations and voluntary organizations at the state level.

The tasks of the state councils are more complex, although perhaps less confusing than those at the national level, since the state organizations tend to create *one* research sub-system which has responsibility for serving as the convenor of meetings of nurse researchers and in general serves the functions performed by both the Council of Nurse Researchers and the Commission on Nursing Research at the national level. State councils can be concerned with providing a mechanism for eventual collaboration among nurse researchers, with cooperation/collaboration between nurse researchers and nurse clinicians. They are concerned with communication networks, with aggrandizing the amount of research being done, with facilitating the conduct of research in the state, and with implementation of research findings into practice. Each state research sub-system must therefore *set priorities* and deal with the prag-matics of tackling certain priorities in the near future and putting other goals off indefinitely. Hopefully, at least a few of the state councils will attempt to influence the relevant state and voluntary agencies in an attempt to make more research monies available for nursing research. The nursing divisions of the state departments of health may or may not be able to support intramural and extramural nursing research at the present time. Physicians head state departments of health and they must be persuaded that nursing research is also needed in the areas of maternal-child health, nursing home care, and chronic disease care. Heretofore, the research thrust has been toward medi-cal research, basic biological research, and medical epidemiology.

At least two different approaches have emerged in the early years of state councils. One approach focuses on potential consumers of research and uses a normative-educative strategy of group processes, study groups, workshops, and conferences to produce more sophisticated research consumers among the state's nurse population. The other approach is to more closely parallel the ANA Council of Nurse Researchers by having membership limited to nurses with at least a master's degree who have been engaged in research or research training. This model focuses largely on having nurse-researchers in different parts of the state get to know each other, with the goal of develop-ing collaborative relationships, research partnerships, cluster studies or research consortia. One of the state councils is attempting to develop strong ties with the Clinical Specialist Council with the hope that researchers and clinicians can become partners in clinical research projects in the future. The Clinical Specialist Council in this state also restricts its membership to master's-prepared nurses with preparation for advanced practice.

A UNITED FRONT THROUGH CONFEDERATION

The bottom line to the foregoing discussion is that several national-, regional-, and state-level groups of nurses are currently involved in promoting research. Some do it directly; others do it indirectly. Unfortunately, each one does it *separately*. If a solid support base for nursing research is to be built, something must be done to amalgamate the fragmented efforts of these numerous groups.

To this end, the ANA Commission on Nursing Research should spearhead an attempt to form some type of confederation that would include: the ANA Commission on Nursing Research, the ANA Council of Nurse Researchers, the American Nurses Foundation, Sigma Theta Tau-Research Fund Committee, the National League for Nursing, the American Association of Colleges of Nursing, and the Principal Investigators and Project Directors Group.* Other groups which may wish to join such a consolidated effort include: the Western Interstate Commission on Nursing, Research Program; the Western Society for Research in Nursing; the Southern Regional Education Board, Council on Collegiate Education for Nursing; the Committee on Institutional Cooperation, Panel on Nursing Education; and perhaps even the state councils.

Organizing such a large number of organizations into a unified confederation would be a formidable task. No one would deny that the opinions would be diverse and the vested interests many. At the same time, a unified position should be obtainable, since these groups have each experienced both the relative powerlessness of nursing in the political arena and the Herculean efforts required to get even a token appropriation for nursing research, or for graduate education in nursing, under the prevailing caste system of the health professions in the United States. A great deal of cooperation and compromise would be required, but the potential payoff could be a new day for nursing research and hence a new day for the object of nursing research: improved health care for the consumer.

Local Level

The local level is usually a specific geographic area composed of certain counties or a region of a state. The population, the square mileage, the nursing resources, the health care facilities, and the educational facilities in local

---

*Three organizations—the AACN, ANA, and NLN—did form an Interorganization Committee for Implementation in 1973. This joint group published a statement in 1973 entitled, "Nursing's Contribution and Commitment." The statement does not contain the word "research," even though the whole thrust of the statement is about nursing's unique contribution to health care services.

nursing organizations differ greatly. This discussion will be skewed toward those with a rich supply of local resources both because it is easier to talk about such areas and because even the most richly endowed areas are not currently taking advantage of their resources to promote nursing research.

The local level nurses association (the district level) will be used as the prototype for discussion here, but any local association of nurses could alter these suggestions to suit their own specific goals. Many groups of nurses with special interests and/or special certifications exist. A few such groups are ostomy nurses, coronary intensive care nurses, renal dialysis nurses, nurse anesthetists, nurse midwives, and so on.

The district nurses associations vary a great deal in their organizational structure in one sense, and are generally alike in another sense. Most of them do have special interest or specialty groups that have program meetings, workshops and the like in addition to the general program meetings for the entire district membership. The district could be operative in supporting research in at least four ways: (1) the district could financially support nursing research by contributing money to local and national nursing research foundations (e.g., local university Nursing Research Development Funds) and to the American Nurses Foundation; (2) it could sponsor short courses on specific research methods or evaluation methods, or it could invite nurse researchers to talk about their projects at program meetings; (3) it could serve the same function as an employing organization, such as a hospital or a college of nursing services, by promulgating specific research interest groups and group studies—this might be done by convincing one or more specialty groups (sections) to engage in action research relative to a specific problem they have identified. Success would require considerable guidance from a local nurse-researcher; or it could be done by organizing a special interest group of nurse-researchers or of people interested in learning either how to conduct or evaluate and use research findings. Finally, (4) the district could serve the influence function at the local level by promoting the funding of nursing research by local family foundations; by the local voluntary associations; by local corporations, businesses, and clubs; and by publicizing through the local media results of nurse-conducted research which would be of interest to the consumer public.

The first two and the fourth suggestions are fairly straight-forward and discussion about them will be brief; the third suggestion will receive somewhat more attention in hopes that progressive districts will want to pursue this suggestion further. Direct financial support for nursing research can go three ways: (1) the district officers can obtain authorization from the membership to make contributions from the treasury; (2) individual district members can be encouraged to make personal contributions which are tax deductible; and (3) contributions can be made indirectly—for example, in memory of a deceased member, or speaker's honoraria can be contributed in the speaker's name and/or the district's name. This latter mechanism is particularly useful as a way to acknowledge the contributions of a speaker who is a member of the district and is thus expected to decline the offer of an honorarium.

It is the author's belief that nurse-researchers who serve as guest speakers should always accept honoraria that they do not wish to keep and specify where it is to be sent as a contribution in their name. This tactic serves more than one purpose. It funnels a tax-deductible contribution into nursing research; it raises the consciousness of the host organization about contributing to nursing research foundations; and it shows the nurse-researcher's personal commitment to supporting with money what was promoted verbally in the speech.* Finally, the district can support research directly by funding specific small projects, or by maintaining a research fund that can be tapped by members or students whose proposals are deemed meritorious.

The second suggestion for district level support relates to the continuing education capability of the district. With the current trend of requiring continuing education credits for license renewal, it seems reasonable that a fair share of the short courses, workshops, and program meetings should be devoted to research in any and all of its phases, including criticism of studies and utilization of findings.

The third suggestion is offered as a way to promote research among nurses employed in organizations where nursing is either a minor component of the system or where research is an unacceptable activity. Nurses that fit these criteria are those in occupational health, in residential clinics for special populations like the aged, in nursing homes, or in residences for exceptional children or adults, (e.g. orphanages, reformatories, penitentiaries, blind schools, deaf schools, or schools for the developmentally disabled). Nurses who work in such settings are rarely encouraged to do research by their employers. Yet nurses in such settings frequently have researchable questions in their heads and access to subjects. Although a particular setting might only employ one or a few nurses, there may be a sizeable group of such nurses that meets under the auspices of the district association. Why not make use of the peer group to translate some question or discomfort about practice into a project? What better way is there to fulfill the concept of a section on practice? The usual evolution of this approach is to have a nurse-researcher speak at a program meeting and then ask the person to serve as a consultant to the group in its planning sessions.

The other alternatives in the third suggestion were about forming new groups within the district. One idea was to form a group of nurse-researchers. This idea may be highly desirable in an area with many researchers in many

*Otherwise known as putting your money where your mouth is.

different organizations and no state council. The idea of forming one or more interest groups concerned with utilization of research could be a highly valuable undertaking. Something like a journal club, or a research utilization review group composed of a mixture of researchers, practitioners, and administrators could have an impact on local service settings by using selected research findings.

The fourth suggestion for the local district was that it use its influence to pave the way for access of nurse-researchers to local sources of research monies. So often the interests of local family foundations are restricted to research done by physicians, although the spirit of the foundations' stated goals would apply equally to research done by either nurses or a multidisciplinary team. Too often physicians and lay persons assume that a multidisciplinary research team means a team made up of something like a surgeon, an internist, an endocrinologist, and a radiologist. A concerted effort by the district could alter this and many other erroneous beliefs that have resulted in the unfair favoritism toward medical research embraced by practically every health/illness-oriented foundation and association in the United States.

ORGANIZATIONAL SUPPORT—STRUCTURE AND STRATEGIES

This section will deal with research support mechanisms that could be built into any employing organization and/or its relevant sub-units. Referrents in this context include: colleges of nursing; schools or departments of nursing; nursing service departments in any type of service agency; and the administrative component in myriad multi-disciplinary service agencies, which employ nurses as professional therapists but do not departmentalize personnel on the basis of disciplinary background—an example would be community mental health centers. The comments and suggestions made here should, if they are sensible and useful for nursing, be equally applicable to other disciplines as well. The following beliefs are presented so the reader will be informed about the framework that serves as the basis for the strategies suggested in this section.

1. A belief that social-structure and social-process are by nature cyclical and reciprocal over time: (a) that a little of each in interaction produces clearer definitions of each; (b) that repeated cycles of influence between structure and process produce a crystallized social entity which has an observable structure and observable patterns of social process; and (c) that the social processes thus produced are congruent with the structure and vice versa.
2. A belief that administrators *can* alter the social-structure/social process cycle, within limits. Limits include: ethical limits, resource limits, time and tolerance limits, and limits determined by the strength and degree of restraining forces.

3. Acceptance of Lewin's change model, which includes three stages: unfreezing, change, and refreezing.[6] Given this change model, there is an identifiable order to the strategies that is useful in effecting change in social systems. The major strategies in order of their suggested application are: (a) consciousness raising; (b) relevant structural reorganization; (c) overt reinforcement of unfreezing signals as they appear in the target groups; (d) creation of new reference groups composed of the early unfreezers and early changers; (e) recycling the products of the early changers back to the more recalcitrant ones; (f) formation of additional new reference groups or integration of second-round unfreezers/changers into the first-round reference groups; (g) the use of clout, power coercion, overt giving of rewards, and overt withholding of rewards on the basis of changing or remaining frozen; (h) maintaining an open invitation to late unfreezers to join the change process; (i) grooming and reinforcing the early unfreezers as partners in stabilizing the change and making it the traditional method; and (j) going deeper into the social fabric of the organization to discover major mismatches, raising the consciousness level about them, and reinforcing moves toward resolving these mismatches.

4. A belief that the three basic ingredients necessary to effect the planned change of integrating research into a nursing system are: (a) at least two people (or one person with access to an outside mentor/advisor) sophisticated in theory and process of planned change; (b) a flexible (small) amount of money with a flexible hand on the purse strings; (c) time, in the sense of relative freedom from artificially set deadlines; and (d) patience—it helps to view the whole process as multiple cycles or rounds of incremental changes, each building toward the major goal in a developmental context.

Planned Change Applied to the Institutionalization of Nursing Research

Initiation of a move by academic or service organizations toward the integration of (nursing) research into their ongoing mission is energized in different ways. For some, the push comes from outside. Examples include special solicitations from funding agencies, accreditation criteria, promotion and tenure criteria, quality assurance, and other evaluation programs. For others the push comes from within, most often but not always led by a newcomer who is usually in an administrative or prestigious staff position. Any of the foregoing can be the "identified" initiating force.*

*Such simplistic causes and effects do not actually occur in social systems, but the simplistic statement is made here to point out that specific antecedents can often be identified as benchmarks in the evolution of change.

Undesirable external pressures can be just as positively influential in over-coming restraining forces as can positively valued external inducements. The converse is also true. To put it more bluntly, *anything* that gets a social system (of nurses) unfrozen and moving toward the research enterprise is worthwhile.

Many persons will, no doubt, disagree with this position. That is under-standable and desirable. In anticipation of such disagreement, the following explication is included in hopes that it will add some substance to the poten-tial debate over conflicting philosophies. In the wake of change, whether planned change, change by drift, or catastrophic change, loss is to be ex-pected. Change cannot occur without loss. It is not possible to add something on which is fundamentally different and simultaneously keep intact what existed before.*

The transformation of the caterpillar into a butterfly seems a useful allegory here. A caterpillar with the features of a butterfly added on would be neither a good caterpillar nor a good butterfuly. The successful change from cater-pillar to butterfly involves loss of parts of the old "self," trust in the urges toward change, major redefinition of the spatial and functional relationship between insect and environment—in other words, a metamorphosis. The caterpillar's change as an allegory corresponds relatively well to the meta-morphosis of nurses into nurse-researchers. A successful change requires loss of, or more accurately, transformations in certain areas of the self-system; trust in the urges toward change and the support system that assists in the process; incrementally experienced major redefinition of the functional and role relationships between the nurse and the environment. So the losses turn out to be paradoxical. They are good losses—the suffering, the anxieties, and the self-doubt are developmental artifacts. Those who would "save" col-leagues from the pains of growth are apparently blind to the long-term dam-age their rescue activities produce.

Specific examples of the application of what is sometimes called "tough love" may help the reader sift through personal attitudes. Very bright young or not-so-young people should be confronted about drifting through their careers with the minimum acceptable amount of educational preparation and concomittant credentials. Drifting along that way is a waste of human potential and indirectly sabotages nursing's brain trust. Persons who do not fulfill criteria for appointment, tenure, or promotion should not be hired, rescued, or kicked-up under the guise of expediency. Soft decisions often

---

*Nurse leaders and nursing groups are extremely prone to this error of incorporating the new by adding it onto the old. This habit has been called "nursing the system" or "nurs-ing the old guard." Such pseudo-nurturing behavior usually ends up sabotaging the change and keeps everybody from growing, especially the shielded "old guard."

mean an underlying cowardice vis-à-vis accepting responsibility for decisions and dealing with the usual backlash. It is a fact that many if not most people who have been given the advantage of "tough love" take stock of their lives and careers, define their personal goals, and go on to pursue them. The major lingering negative feeling that they do continue to express seems to be embarrassment or wounded pride because they did not have the personal foresight to see themselves and their career trajectories in a clearer light by themselves. Eventually they may even come to accept and forgive themselves for this very human oversight.

There are a few strategies useful in integrating research into the social fabric of an organization which have received short shrift in the foregoing discussion. One important strategy is change in the formal structure of an organization or relevant sub-unit. If research is truly to become integrated in an organization, then it must be accorded bureaucratic power and a high level of visibility vis-à-vis the ongoing business of that organization. Structural changes in this context include changes in the table or organization, changes in the way that formal communication and authority lines are laid out, and changes in the composition of administration vis-à-vis *what* gets defined as meriting an administrative head. There are at least two conflicting camps on the issue of whether it is better for a change agent to be an unobtrusive member of the staff, by holding a staff position with no administrative power, or whether it is better for a change agent to be in an administrative position. The reader should understand that this author believes the administrative route to have a higher probability of success.*

Those organizations which are serious about integrating research into their basic mode of operations would do well to give serious attention to altering the formal structure of their organization, so that there is a match between the goal and basic operations of the organization.

At the Ohio State University School of Nursing, research development efforts went on for about 12 years at a tangential enterprise that had no formal links to the reward system in the school.[7] People who did not do research and did not publish in scholarly journals were promoted or tenured for other activities, such as committee service. The research development enterprise was an ad hoc enterprise. The project director had no say in top level decisions made by the Executive Committee. Quite often Executive Commitee decisions competed with the Research Development Program for

*This belief in administratively based change agency represents a shift in opinion based on multiple observations of aborted planned change efforts in hospitals, nursing homes, and health centers. In every instance, the change agents who held those staff positions were well trained, appropriately credentialed, knowledgeable people. Conversely, the author has observed successfully implemented and integrated planned change efforts when the credentialed change agent was in an administrative position.

faculty time and attention. Hence, the decision-makers were unwittingly undermining the research support process.

The Ohio State University School of Nursing faculty made a well thought through series of structural changes to remedy this condition in 1973. These changes consisted of adding an assistant director for research and making the research committee a standing committee of the school. Thus the research enterprise was accorded administrative importance equal to the Undergraduate Program, the Graduate Program, Continuing Education, and Student Affairs, each of which was headed by an assistant director on the Table of Organization.

There are disadvantages to the administrative-line approach. They can be grossly subsumed under two categories: (1) negative attitudes toward administrators, and (2) time-consuming administrative rituals. The advantages are many and even include the disadvantages just listed—again, there is the paradox of disadvantages becoming advantages.

When a clear commitment to research is evidenced in a table or organization, the scene is set for nurturing a self-fulfilling prophecy. The prophecy is that the employing organizations, i.e., the school or health agency, highly values and firmly supports research and researchers. The fact that this is a myth in the early period is irrelevant. The more people come to believe in the myth and act as if it were true, the less of a myth it becomes. Eventually, the organization as a social system acts as if it does in fact highly value and firmly support research and researchers. At that point it becomes merely an academic exercise to determine whether the commitment is fake or real. The system is behaving as if it were committed.[8]

Centralized Research Resources

A number of organizations have been engaged in research development long enough to have a well developed track record and a cadre of researchers on their staff who can be counted on to have either projects in process or proposals in preparation most of the time. Such organizations usually find it more efficient to develop a centralized locus for the administration and facilitation of the business end of the research process. The centralized research locus may serve as a business office with an administrative assistant to coordinate personnel appointments, purchasing, and so on. It may take on the dimension of a professional service by having one or more consultants and technicians available to help investigators. It may become an identifiable entity in its own right, for instance a research center or institute.

R. Louise McManus directed the first such centralized facility in nursing. It was organized in 1953 at Teachers College, Columbia University and was called the Institute of Research and Service in Nursing Education. The purpose of this institute related primarily to nursing education and educational research. The first centralized resource dedicated to nursing research per se was founded at Wayne State University College of Nursing in 1969. Harriet H. Werley was its first director.[9] The Ohio State University (OSU) School of Nursing was the site of the second center for nursing research, which began in 1972.[10] There are disadvantages to a separate center identity such as potential isolation of nursing faculty or students who are the very people most essential to the center's purpose. Other organizations are just beginning the research development process and have not yet built up the consistent demand for predictable resources (people-resources, supplies, equipment, etc.) that can most efficiently be handled through centralization.

There are several universities which operate a nursing research office which serves several of the same pragmatic and educational functions as a center. However, the traditional concept of a research center in academe is broader in purpose. Centers may define their constituency to include not only faculty in the specific college or school, but also graduate students, exceptionally bright undergraduate students, members of other relevant disciplines, and practitioners, faculty, and students from other settings within a designated geographic area served by the center.

Each type of centralized facility can be supportive to nursing research by being supportive of nurse-researchers. Planning, coordination, and evaluation of formal and informal strategies to this end are usually handled by the person or persons who head up the research office or center. The judicious allocation of seed money, money to cover inflation or unforeseen costs in funded research, can all be handled through the research office, with decision-making about budgetary allocation in the hands of a group of competent persons.

A total process approach is being attempted, within certain pragmatic limits, at the OSU Center for Nursing Research. This support strategy might be called the "fairy godmother" approach. The assumption underlying this service program is that investigators are extremely busy with teaching and service. The little time they have available to do research is precious and it should be used for research, not for the administrative trivia that surrounds research projects in bureaucratic organizations. To this end, the core staff has been chosen and/or trained to interface between the researcher and other people or things: (1) core staff members advertise for and do a preliminary screen of research assistants and other technical staff, set up interviews with the investigator, and then process all the paperwork for the appointments when the investigator decides who is to be hired; (2) general consultants are hired, by the year or on an hourly fee-for-actual-use basis—consultants in research design, statistical analysis, computer programming, and manuscript editing are on call to investigators, and appointments can be set up by a core staff member; (3) core staff members process orders for supplies and equipment; (4) they run errands to the central campus, libraries, computer centers, and the research foundation; (5) a core secretary types and duplicates, gets required signatures, and mails; (6) core research assistants train data collectors under the supervision of the investigator, and advise on pragmatics about data collection; (7) these assistants help set up coding formats and procedures, and train coders to follow these procedures and acceptable methods of verification; and (8) core research assistants search for consultants in specific areas of expertise needed on a given project, set up appointments, and handle other matters at the interface.

The core consultants can come to the consultee so the nurse-investigator does not have to spend time in travel to the consultant's office and back. The other services are also set up so that as many as possible of the frustrating and time-consuming bureaucratic details which go with modern-day research can be handled by experienced staff members who know the system and who have become expert at working with it. This strategy greatly enhances the investigator's capacity to use time allocated to research efficiently, by anticipating his or her needs for common resources and services and having them easily accessible and convenient to use.

Neophyte researchers using university or school funds usually make use of many of these services. Seasoned researchers with larger external grants usually use the center in the early phases before funding, later to orient their project staff, and sporadically for services not built into their grant budgets.

Overall, this approach has been successful in achieving its purpose. Furthermore, the cost of the operation is minimal.

PEER SUPPORT—STRUCTURE AND STRATEGIES

Orchestrating a peer support system is the most exciting and rewarding of all the strategies discussed in this chapter. When two or more neophytes begin to hear each other and to experience the phenomena of sisterhood, guided by a seasoned research mentor, the outcomes can go beyond anyone's expectations. Peer support groups work in somewhat the same way as self-help groups. The entire group shares in the responsibility for teaching, criticising, bolstering, correcting, or praising the other members vis-à-vis the development or conduct of that person's research project. Myriad variations of peer support groups are possible. The Western Interstate Commission of Higher Education in Nursing (WICHEN) uses a variation wherein several people from the western states interested in one research problem develop their proposal so that each member will be responsible for implementing the design with a sample in their home state. In effect, these are consortia with multiple simultaneous replications.

Another variation is to form a group around a topic of special interest. The common elements of the topic, i.e., theories, research, and literature on content, can be reviewed and discussed early in the group's existence. Later, individuals, dyads, or other self-selected groupings determine specific research problems they wish to pursue. The group then becomes a medium for testing out the stages of the proposal-writing process and later an encouragement system during the implementation, analysis, and reporting phases. These groups should not be dissolved too early. A neophyte researcher needs support during the later phases of implementation just as much as during the planning stages.

Additional indirect benefits accrue from peer support groups. New friendships, colleague relationships, and cliques form. These relationships help to compensate for any pejorative feedback coming from anti-research peers. They also serve to decrease the sense of isolation experienced by researchers. Finally, the proposals that emanate from these groups have been worked and reworked. They contain the thinking of many people, but the decisions and written narrative of one or two, or of a small team. Proposals generated through this mechanism should be clearer and more internally consistent than proposals written by one or two persons in relative isolation.

Certainly not all peer support groups are successful. Sometimes the aggregate of people who self-select into the group do not gel with each other or with the mentor/facilitator. Other times, there is a mixture of reasons for joining the group—some want to produce a study, others want to be participant-observers in the group sessions but do not want to work toward developing research projects themselves. It is up to the mentor/facilitator and the group members to assess the progress of the group from time to time and to make sensible decisions about whether to disband, reorganize, or keep going the same way. A useful rule of thumb is to expect about 30 to 40 percent of peer support groups to be productive. Expect a few more groups to have a few productive members. Expect about 30 to 40 percent of the groups to disband for any of several valid reasons. The major point to remember is that when a peer support group flops, do not consider it a failure of the peer group concept. Wait a few months and organize another peer group some other way. Orient the next group to the fact that some trials and errors may be necessary until a comfortable mix of people find each other and can get down to work.

Individual Level

Individual nurses are where the buck stops vis-à-vis support for and development of nursing research as a social institution. The individual nurse is the target and must either accept or reject whatever support is offered from the environment.

Individual nurses support the research potential in themselves by taking courses in theory development, research methods, instrument development, statistics, evaluation methods, and technical writing. They support nursing research by being receptive to development efforts on their behalf.

Young nurses who show promise in those cognitive and psychomotor dimensions usually associated with successful research performance ought to be identified early in their undergraduate program and introduced to real live nurse-researchers. Research assistantships, group studies, and independent studies are useful mechanisms to get young undergraduate and early graduate students involved in a research project that is not too much for them to handle.

Neophyte nurse-researchers benefit greatly from the traditional mode of apprenticeship with one or more mentors. Apprenticeship was frowned upon as a method for training nurse researchers until very recently. Apparently the fear of being accused of exploiting students for personal gain was the basis for rejecting it as a method. The alternative approach, wherein every student is expected to generate, conduct, and report on a study of his or her own, has not proved to be an acceptable substitute. It serves to maintain the students' civil rights, but robs them of the benefits to be derived from participating in a study directed by a competent researcher. In recent years, increasing numbers of nurses with doctoral preparation in the biological and behavioral sciences have brought back into nursing the research-mentor tradition which is so strong in those sciences. This tradition has always carried the potential threat of abuse, but the dangers are far outweighted by the benefits that accrue from the role modeling that occurs.

In the past, federal traineeships for graduate study in nursing and some pre-doctoral fellowships have excluded part-time employment of students. In many cases, this has had the paradoxical effect of keeping the brightest students out of part-time jobs as research assistants. In the future, regulations should be written in such a way that research assistantships are not excluded. Unhappily, a whole generation of master's students has been excluded from significant amounts of participation in their mentors' research projects.

Neophytes and potential nurse-researchers cannot be supported unless they accept the support and do their half of the development work. Nobody can make anybody else into something they do not wish to become. Honest communication on both sides saves everybody's time and energy and cuts down on frustration. Persons who do not want to be "developed" as researchers should say so. The would-be developers should respect each nurse's right to make decisions about his or her own future. The principle of readiness applies here: some nurses are just not ready. Leave them alone for awhile and let them experience life a little longer. Many of them do get interested in higher levels of education and preparation for a research career if they are not coerced at the improper time.

Credentialed nurse-researchers with a track record of external support and self confidence about their research knowledge may go through periods of nonproductivity in research. Teaching workloads or curriculum changes may become too burdensome. Some researchers move into administrative positions, some become exhausted with the frantic pace of leading three or four lives, some become ill, and some need time to mull over the ramifications of their research findings in order to develop some logical synthesis before developing a new study. Some researchers have exhausted a specific avenue of research and others have become disinterested in a specific area of research—either way, such people need time to talk, think, and become comfortable with where they want to go in future research efforts.

The peer support group mechanism is sometimes a successful strategy to use with seasoned researchers as well as with neophyte researchers. The group meetings are different in content and operation but the underlying benefits are about the same. The tired and haggard seasoned researchers derive remotivation and increased energy to think new thoughts and get excited about new avenues of research in the peer group atmosphere.

INFORM, INFLUENCE, AND INFILTRATE

This chapter has contained numerous admonitions to organized nursing to increase the clout of nursing as compared to medicine and others vying for the research dollar and other requisite resources. In this section on the individual level, it is appropriate to make suggestions about what a single nurse-researcher can do to influence the support base for nursing research. A three-step strategy is proposed which might be called the "Three In-System." First nurses can inform the consumer public and the policy/law-makers about nursing research—what it is, what it does, how it is useful, what happens to its products, who can do it, where it can be done, and what resources are required to do it.

Next, the public, the members of the more powerful professions, the legislators, the bureaucrats, and the decision-makers in private foundations must hear about nursing research over and over again. There must be intermittent reinforcements about the values of nursing research in order to *influence* these people and to counteract, in at least a small way, the influence exerted by other professions over several decades.

Third, nurses must get onto more boards and executive committees of funding agencies, foundations, and voluntary organizations. One of the reasons that it is so easy for medical researchers to get funded is that the HEW study sections, the foundation boards, and the boards of the voluntary associations are all packed with physicians. It is easier to read and approve proposals in one's own field because the jargon is familiar and many of the methods are standard. Hence, even a poorly written proposal by a physician can be understood. Gaps in the written design are assumed to be oversights. Not so when the proposal is being reviewed by members of another discipline. The terms, the methods, and the underlying theories are foreign, so the gaps cannot be filled in with assumptions based on the investigator's credentials. Therefore the proposal is rejected. If more nurses were appointed to more positions as peer reviewers, as high-level federal bureaucrats, as members of foundation boards, and as members of the boards and peer review groups of voluntary associations like the American Cancer Society and the American Heart Association, they could more adequately review and translate nursing proposals to the rest of the reviewers.

The strategy to *infiltrate* a voluntary association goes like this: (1) volunteer at the local level, go to meetings, talk at meetings and make yourself known to members after the meeting; (2) become a member of a committee, become the chairperson of a committee, run for or get appointed to the board of directors; (3) solicit proposals from competent nurse-researchers and work until that organization gets used to funding nurse investigators; (4) meanwhile, get active at the next higher level—the state level, for example— and go through the whole process over again.

If possible, groom several younger colleagues to follow behind you each step of the way, so that the gains can be held and even improved. It is also useful to get nurses moving up through associations in neighboring regions and neighboring states so that executive directors of these associations become aware that it is a wide-spread trend. Eventually it becomes an okay thing for nurses to be in responsible positions in an association and for the association to fund nurse-investigators. All this can follow from the actions of one nurse-researcher.

SUMMARY

The position taken in this chapter has been that support for nursing research should go from the national level to the grass roots level and back up again. National organizations are encouraged to concentrate their confederated influence on national-level targets such as the federal government, the big foundations, and the national offices of voluntary associations. Likewise, the regional, state, and local level nursing groups are encouraged to concentrate their influences toward the goal of promoting nursing research throughout the geographic area they serve. The national organizations would thus be able to call on the regional, state, and local organizations vis-à-vis communication to individual congressmen and expect a well-organized response on short notice.

The employing organization is the most important link in the chain from the national level down to the individual nurse-researcher. An organization that avidly supports research will show research productivity among its nurses no matter what is or is not happening elsewhere. An organization which is apathetic, naive, or antagonistic to research will have little or no research in process, regardless of the opportunities and resources extant in the environment. This chapter's discussion about support of nursing research and nurse-researchers within organizations refers to any place that employs or educates nurses.

In those organizations where only one or a few nurses are employed and where research is feasible but not the norm for employees, it is suggested that the local nurses association serve as the catalytic agent to foster specific research projects in problem areas of interest to this group. Besides a willing nurse staff, a second crucial component would be access to a state council of nurse-researchers or a local nurse-researcher willing to serve as a consultant to the team.

The peer group process has been discussed at some length in this chapter. The responsibilities individual nurses have to be receptive to research development activities on their behalf was also discussed, along with the major educational strategies that are useful for training researchers. Finally, a three-step strategy was presented that individual nurses can use to effect large system support for nursing research.

REFERENCES

1. E.P. McGriff, "The Courage for Effective Leadership in Nursing," *Image* 8 (October 1976): 56-60.
2. L. Noe (ed.), *The Foundation Grants Index,* 1972 ed. (New York: Columbia University Press, 1973).
3. R.G. Campos, "Securing Information on Funding Sources for Nursing Research," *Journal of Nursing Administration* 6 (October 1976): 16-18.
4. R. Chow, *Identifying Nursing Action with the Care of Postoperative Cardiac Patients* (Columbus, Ohio: Ohio State University Research Foundation, 1967).
5. L.E. Notter and A.F. Spector, *Nursing Research in the South, A Survey,* Collegiate Education for Nursing Report of 21st Meeting (Atlanta: Southern Regional Education Board Council on Collegiate Education for Nursing, 1974).
6. K. Lewin, *Field Theory in Social Science* (New York: Harper, 1951).
7. J.S. Stevenson, *Research Development Program in Nursing* (Columbus, Ohio: Ohio State University Research Foundation, 1975).
8. H.S. Becker, "Personal Change in Adult Life," in B.L. Neugarten (ed.), *Middle Age and Aging* (Chicago: University of Chicago Press, 1968).

9. H.H. Werley and F.P. Shea, "The First Center for Research in Nursing," *Nurs Res* 22 (May–June 1973): 217–31.
10. J.S. Stevenson, *Research Development Program in Nursing* (Columbus, Ohio: Ohio State University Research Foundation, 1975).

BIBLIOGRAPHY

Diers, D. "Faculty Research Development at Yale," *Nurs Res* 19: 64–71, January–February 1970.

Felton, G., and McLaughlin, F.E. "The Collaborative Process in Generating a Nursing Research Study," *Nurs Res* 25: 115–20, March–April 1976.

The Robert Wood Johnson Foundation. *Annual Report 1975.* Princeton, New Jersey, 1975.

Sanazaro, P.J. "Federal Health Services R & D Under the Auspices of the National Center for Health Services Research and Development." In Flook E.E., and Sanazaro, P.J., eds.). *Health Services Research and R & D in Perspective.* Ann Arbor: Health Administration Press, 1973, 150–83.

Schlotfeldt, R.M. *Creating a Climate for Nursing Research.* Cleveland, Ohio: Frances Payne Bolton School of Nursing, Case Western Reserve University, 1973.

Shirk, F.I. *Developing Competency of Nursing Faculty in Research.* Columbus, Ohio: Ohio State University Research Foundation, 1970.

Voda, A.M., Butts, S.V., and Gress, L.D. "On the Process of Involving Nurses in Research." *Nurs Res* 20: 302–8, July–August 1971.

CHAPTER FOUR

CLINICAL AND THEORETICAL RESEARCH

Florence S. Downs

Professional communities sustain themselves through a set of shared, generalized beliefs about the nature and best implementation of their respective missions. These notions may be derived from a number of sources, such as tradition, historical accident, contemporary values, and deliberate investigation. As a group moves to establish greater autonomy as a profession, concomitant efforts are made to define the unique characteristics and functions that enable the group to offer a valued service. Since appeals to tradition or personal experience lack persuasive credibility as evidence, it follows that deliberate examination, which is governed by a set of rules that command attention, will increase.

Kuhn points out that "Failure of existing rules is the prelude to the search for new ones."[1] The emphasis in nursing for some time has been that the new rules are those which govern the scientific enterprise, since it is from these that a critical mass of defensible nursing knowledge is most likely to arise. An explicit statement concerning this issue was made by the House of Delegates of the American Nurses' Association in 1974:

WHEREAS, nursing is a discipline in need of further developing and testing its body of knowledge, and

WHEREAS, the communication of nursing knowledge would be enhanced by the existence of tested concepts and constructs, and

WHEREAS, research is one of the primary means of documenting the efficiency and effectiveness of practice, and

WHEREAS, nursing lacks significant influence, power, and prestige because of its inability to specify its contribution to health care; therefore be it

RESOLVED, that the American Nurses' Association make a concerted effort to build a public image of nursing research as an essential contribution to knowledge in the health care field, and be it further

RESOLVED, that during the next decade the principal thrust of nursing to be a threefold one, namely

a. the development of systematically derived information relevant to the practice of nursing,

b. the development and testing of theories in practice,

c. document the outcomes and effectiveness of practice.[2]

In addition to documenting the emphasis on the "new rules," the preceding statement points out other interesting and often ignored features associated with an increase in research activity: the close link between the use of scientific methodology and the establishment of professional credibility, influence, and power; and the ability to create and foster a new public image.

Throughout the ensuing discussion it would be well to keep the foregoing in mind. The intent here is not to undercut the crucial role of research in the improvement of health, but to point out that in reality research tends to be viewed in terms that are hardly neutral. The words *progress, advancement,* and *betterment* are recurrent qualifiers. (My use of the word *improvement* is a prime example.) It may be that the *process* of research, in itself, is value free, but the questions chosen for exploration may not be. Indeed, they are often closely tied to social priorities and the disciplinary philosophies of the times. Even a cursory inspection of the funding patterns of the federal government will show that monies for investigation are apportioned with an eye to the needs of the nation, whether for health, space exploration, or warfare. Considering the immense amounts of financial resources the government has poured, and continues to pour, into research efforts, it is not at all surprising that there is a trend toward increased specification of the nature of scientific endeavor.

Further, in mature sciences the questions for which answers are sought are embedded in the educational milieu. That is to say, the direction of scientific effort is determined by a set of knowns and unknowns inculcated by educational leaders who are themselves dedicated scientists. Both student and teacher are part of a scientific community that consumes the same literature and shares the same goals. This process tends to ensure an orderly transmission of current theory and knowledge, socializes the student into the arena of important problems in the field, and points out the likely methodology required for the solution of these problems.

Nursing exemplifies in many ways the stages of self-examination and inquiry through which an occupation must pass on its way to professionalization. We are almost beyond the questions related to the nature of the group and its functions: "Who or what are we?" "What do we do differently from others, and how can we do it better?" The answers to these queries have helped to define the boundaries of nursing, and they provide a base from which a set of questions appropriate to the field may be determined. It would appear we have begun to enter into the next stage—there is a recognized need for knowledge through which practice decisions can be postulated, and for information to determine precisely which phenomena are of concern to the discipline. Although the questions "What is research?" and, more specifically, "What is research in nursing?" have been raised for a long time, this new phase of development will take the answers beyond mere rhetoric to an actual shaping of tomorrow's research-related questions, and of nursing's future dimensions.

THE RELATION BETWEEN RESEARCH
AND EVALUATION

In an effort to delineate the difference between research and evaluation, the author surveyed a number of sources and attempted to synthesize a definition of research that would appear, at least on the surface, satisfactory to our immediate purpose. The conclusion was that research is essentially a rational process that tests the presumed relation between phenomena by systematic and objective methods. It is a deliberate procedure, inextricably bound to either the testing of theory or a theoretical rationale. As we shall later see, it is only when the definition of research is teamed with a desired or valued practice outcome that there is substantial room for argument.

The converse is true of the term *evaluation*. As long as evaluation is framed within the context of its goal, its definition is reasonably clear. The explanations of Deming, that "evaluation is a pronouncement concerning the effectiveness of some treatment or plan that has been tried or put into effect,"[3] and Suchman, that evaluation is essentially a process of judging the worth of some activity regardless of the method applied,[4] are definitions that lend themselves to succinct conceptualization. The matter is not so easily managed, however, when the term *research* is appended to evaluation, so that both the process and the outcome are linked, as in the following definition:

"By objective and systematic methods, evaluation research assesses the extent to which goals are realized and looks at the factors associated with successful or unsuccessful outcomes."[5]

The importance of the distinction between research and evaluation would be merely dialectical if both were similarly associated with professional responsibility and accountability. The notions of research and evaluation both encompass the steps of logical decision-making. However, the act of research is ordinarily conceived as one that is value-free, in the sense that the prime focus is on verifying the chain of relations among variables that are essentially "neutral," abstract, and impersonal. As the preceding definitions of evaluation point out rather well, qualitative notions of worth, success, and effectiveness form a large part of the picture. As a result, they cannot be separated from standards of practice, whether the activity is nursing, education, or some other discipline related to effecting change. Research is, of course, to some extent associated with standards of practice. But research determines the content of the knowledge or input on which practice is based, and it is unnecessary for all practitioners to possess and utilize research skills as such. Evaluation seeks to appraise the outcomes of practice and consequently should be well within the capabilities of all clinicians.

Some of the uneasy connections between the two processes can be resolved by placing emphasis on the techniques of research as they apply to evaluation, rather than trying to explain evaluation as a special case falling within the rubric of research. As such, evaluation tends to suffer in comparison as a procedure. "*That*'s not *research!*" Zimmer makes this point well:

> Another conflict within the profession arises through use of criteria for research to judge the merits of an evaluation program. To meet requirements of the organization that are shaping the program that is being discussed, staffs in nursing services are implementing *evaluation programs*. These are not clinical research programs. This distinction is important. The purpose is to evaluate nursing practice through use of predetermined, locally defined, and/or accepted standards for criterion variables that are important and specific to a particular patient population. In evaluation, the criterion variables and standards for efficacy are established and known *prior* to the study. These are drawn from the best information available; this includes the results of clinical research.[6]

She further supports this argument with a quotation from Goran *et al.*, which states that in clinical research, "efficacy is not known; it is the variable under study."[7] It can probably be said that far too much investigation which should properly be considered evaluation has been permitted to be labeled as clinical research, thus creating considerable confusion about the distinction between the two processes. Theoretical rationales notwithstanding, if the primary goal is to decide whether one intervention is more effective than another in bringing about a desired outcome, the process is properly referred to as evaluation. A parallel clinical research question is differently phrased. It asks whether there is a relation between one or more interventions and a specific outcome. If more than one intervention is involved, it may also ask whether or not there appears to be a difference in the strength of their association with the dependent variable. The determination of the question related to evaluation may require *experimental methodology* in order to acquire an adequate answer, but the answer to a clinical question requires *experimentation,* and the implications for patients who are participants are clearly dissimilar.

THE NATURE OF THE NURSING PROCESS

Before proceeding into a discussion of the nature of nursing research, it seems prudent to place the set of actions that have come to be referred to as "nursing process" in perspective. This particular terminology seems to have originated sometime in the mid-1960s and has come to be defined as "an orderly, systematic manner of determining the client's problems, making plans to solve them, initiating the plan or assigning others to implement it, and evaluating the extent to which the plan was effective in resolving the problems identified."[8] At the risk of oversimplification, then, nursing process is essentially a decision-oriented procedure, which aims to collect data for a nursing diagnosis and for subsequent interventions that will affect a client's well-being. Given this definition, nursing process is easily distinguished from research, which aims to enhance the knowledge base from which decisions are made, and from evaluation, which illuminates effectiveness against a set of generalized criteria.

NURSING RESEARCH

Since enthusiasm for nursing research seems to be increasing, it seems safe to say that a large segment of the nursing profession ascribes to the notion that research is essential for professional survival. Most nurses agree that nursing practice should be postulated from a knowledge base formed through scientific methods. Most would also agree that our present fund of information is often inadequate and that knowledge directly taken from other disciplines frequently fails to answer nursing questions with any degree of precision. It would be more difficult to obtain a consensus on just what kind of information constitutes a professional base for practice, and consequently on what can be safely labeled as nursing research.

Part of the predicament evolves from different conceptions of which elements compose or should compose the body of knowledge described as nursing science. The whole area tends to be further vitiated by a side argument about whether or not nursing is a basic or an applied science. This is an interesting semantic concern that can incite lively discussion, but it is superfluous to a discussion of the appropriate content of nursing research, at least in its present state of development. The likelihood is that, at some later date, an examination of what has become nursing science through nursing research will yield a rather unequivocal answer to the question. In Johnson's words:

> Sciences, then, become differentiated from one another on the basis of what is studied and the perspective used to raise questions, make observations, and interpret evidence. Since several sciences may, and often do, study the same phenomenon, it is the distinctive perspective of each science which most clearly discriminates it from others. Emergence of the now recognized and accepted basic disciplines is an historical product, brought about by the more or less arbitrary decisions of investigators, as phenomena for study were selected and the particular questions to be asked were identified.[9]

To illustrate the above point, one might consider the condition of alcoholism, which has been studied within sociological, psychological, and physiological contexts. The various treatment regimens prescribed reflect the orientation of the discipline called upon to institute the intervention. Indeed, even within such disciplines there may be variations, determined by research evidence produced by different schools of thought.

In discussions of the proper scope of nursing research, one often hears the words "knowledge borrowed from other fields" to describe some particular facet of nursing science. In the final analysis, there are no divisions of knowledge in the real world. It is we who delineate certain areas of information as "belonging" to certain fields. The possessors of knowledge are those persons who understand it and are aware of how to make use of it in appropriate and creative ways. Basic research in one field may be applied in another, or basic research in several fields may be combined in unique ways to answer a different or expanded set of questions, which questions form the basic research of another or new field.

The position taken here is that the content of nursing science will, in all probability, be derived from two research contexts. One of these is a "basic" component that describes the logical or knowledge base of the discipline, and the other is a more applied focus that explains the functional or professional aspects of nursing service. It should be obvious that the two cannot be dichotomized except for the purpose of discussion. Nonetheless, they present different approaches to the search for knowledge in nursing, approaches that need to be understood within their own frames of reference.

Readers of nursing literature are urged to resist the implication of various authors that the science of nursing will develop from research derived exclusively from nursing practice. This tendency is hard to avoid since nursing first developed as a clinical practice based largely on tradition and experience, and is now attempting to find knowledge to back up that practice. Further, most of us are imbued with a practice orientation that is hard to escape. The conscious or unconscious bias, then, is to twist research knowledge, which is pivotal to the conceptualization of nursing goals, toward a practice orientation. Sharp makes some perceptive observations as concerns our orientation to the behavioral scientist:

> The difference in mode of entrance into their respective professions seemed to be directly related to the respondent's perception of the place of research in nursing. Behavioral scientists perceived research as basic to knowledge and knowledge as basic to practice. Nurses seemed to perceive research as adjunctive to practice and knowledge, but not necessarily fundamental and basic. Whereas the behavioral scientists typically approached problems by first considering the applicability of research knowledge or theory derived from research, the nurses tended to look for solutions both in implications from previous practice patterns and in research and knowledge derived therefrom . . . the nurse who could point to a long period of practice experience with a problem thus seemed to have a status advantage and other nurses tended to appreciate and value this experiential background.[10]

An interesting case in point can be found in an article by Andreoli and Thompson, which discusses the views of Johnson, Rogers, and Gortner, among others, in relation to the content of nursing science.[11] Both Johnson and Rogers write from their interest in the abstract phenomena that characterize the central themes or goals of nursing as a profession. Johnson states as follows:

> It is proposed here that the body of knowledge called the science of nursing consists of a synthesis, reorganization, or extension of concepts drawn from the basic and other applied sciences which in their reformulation tend to become "new" concepts. These concepts will lead to the development of theories of nursing intervention which will yield predictable responses in patients when implemented in nursing care.[12]

Roger's position is similar in this regard, but her prime emphasis is on the identification of indices which reflect the wholeness of the person, as the central focus of nursing, in simultaneous interaction with the environment. Her notion is that these conceptualizations, although certainly related to existing scientific knowledge, will be more than a synthesis and will go beyond available explanatory principles to constitute a new kind of knowledge unique to the domain of nursing.[13]

Gortner and others[14-16] clearly approach the nature of nursing science from a different direction. Gortner states, "Nursing research, in brief, is a systematic inquiry into the problems encountered in nursing practice and into the modalities of patient care, such as support and comfort, prevention of trauma, promotion of recovery, health education, health appraisal, and coordination of health care." In the same article she further emphasizes her position: "Note the key words: patient and effect. This is the critical nucleus of patient care research, of nursing research, of practice for any profession."[14]

It seems clear that the position of Rogers and Johnson is vastly different from that of Gortner in regard to the source of research data that needs to be tapped in order to develop a science of nursing. Yet Andreoli and Thompson deduce that the verifiable knowledge will be derived in either case from nursing practice.[11] Their conclusion is easily traced to the assumption that the term *science of nursing* can in all cases be translated as science originating from the *practice* of nursing.

The crucial point here is that one of the ways to understand some of the diversity in research orientations and interests that presently exists in nursing is to recognize that there is more than one point of departure for equally valid investigations. In time, it is likely that the two positions will become entwined. Practice problems that deal with clinical phenomena, such as intervention in situations involving dying and death, and effective strategies for dealing with pain or life crisis, may finally yield effective answers only after analysis from a highly theoretical perspective. Theoretical problems that seek to explain the nature of the phenomena that constitute nursing as a branch of learning may require clinical trials for full elucidation.

In contemplating the outcomes of such a grand scheme it would be unrealistic to believe that controversy about nursing science would cease. Science has no palpable "body." Its contours are constantly in a state of flux. The chips in the game of science are problems, not facts.

The power of science is in the fluidity it retains through the process of research. Problems and questions are science, not facts and answers. Speaking from the perspective of a scientist, Holton writes, "In truth, each of us who has done something in science treasures these memorable periods of individual euphoria *when one has found a problem*—one that may be tormenting in its complexity, all too slow to crack open—but at least one that promises to be *solvable*, and worthy of throwing one's whole being into."[17] Obviously, research is not viewed as a frivolous activity of the scientist, or as one that can be carried out on a spare-time basis.

Perhaps the best answer to the query "What is nursing research?" is "A good question."

CLASSIFICATION OF RESEARCH
AS THEORETICAL OR APPLIED

Any attempt to discuss the classification or relative merits of theoretical research vis-à-vis clinical or applied research is immediately confronted with the problem of definition. Efforts to resolve this dilemma carry with them the risks of entering into futile debate on the "real importance" of either activity, thus introducing even more confusion into the field. The problem is further compounded by the fact that the mention of theoretical research evokes notions of unreality, rat studies, white coats, laboratories, exquisite control of variables, and an abundance of subtle statistical analyses. In actuality, the experimental method, which is one of the main tools of theoretical research, should be evaluated primarily from the standpoints of the richness of the information it yields, the significance of the conclusions it may reach, and the substance of the hypotheses it generates relative to its theoretical basis.

It should be noted that the use of the world "clinical" as a synonym for "applied" can lead one even further afield. There is really no necessary connection between them. Either theoretical or applied research may be carried out in a clinical setting. An example drawn from Brunner[18] in a discussion of informational sufficiency illustrates this point well: Both a clinician and an experimentalist are interested in finding out what areas of the brain mediate intact pattern vision. The experimentalist goes about finding an answer by systematically blocking various areas of the brain and observing the results in the strict pattern dictated by the rules of science. The clinician, on the other hand, takes cases as they come and tests for brain damage and pattern vision. The attack on the problem is markedly different and the decisions that follow are likely to be different as well. However, there is a rather remarkable similarity in the situations of the two investigators relative to the information sought.

Crowley[19] believes that the core problem in differentiating between "pure" and "applied" research is essentially one of moving from understanding and explaining to the work of predicting and using. She points out that the ultimate distinction between them is really a matter of whether the problem is formulated in terms of its cognitive significance (pure research) or its practical significance within the field of application.

In the first issue of *Nursing Research,* Genevieve Bixler provided as classic a definition of pure and applied research as exists anywhere:

> The term pure research has characterized systematic investigation which is undertaken without consideration of needs and their ultimate satisfaction, for the pleasures to be found in the intellectual pursuit of learning and the accretion of knowledge. The rigid application of logic and the step by step progress from the early unfolding of ideas through the intermediate processes of gathering facts, developing hypotheses, testing and verifying, to reaching conclusions has constituted reason enough for doing. Applied research, on the other hand, develops from problems, from some dislocation in life situations, from a need which is recognized. It is frankly utilitarian. Its objectives are certain to include some which are intended to improve conditions. Change is inherent in the planning when research is the applied sort, for on the bases of the conclusions reached, something is very likely to be changed.[20]

Despite the seeming comprehensiveness of the preceding definition, Cronbach and Suppes[21] do not believe that it solves the classification problem. In *Research for Tomorrow's Schools* they cite as an example the case of the curious monk who cross-fertilized peas, in contrast with the seed company that employs cross-fertilization methods for profit.

The following news release is an excellent demonstration of the previous distinction:

A new crystalline material, not found in nature and never before produced in the laboratory, has been synthesized by scientists in Bell Labs. The new material—named a monolayer crystal—was assembled atomic layer by atomic layer through a crystal growing process called molecular beam epitaxy. It is the first synthetic crystal in which the chemical composition of each atomic layer has been individually controlled.

The material is similar to crystals used in light-emitting diodes and tiny solid-state lasers now under investigation for possible future use in Bell System telecommunications systems. However, the monolayer crystal has new electronic and optical properties. . . . This new crystal growth achievement could permit tailor-making materials with specific, built-in electronic, optical and mechanical properties.[22]

Cronbach and Suppes[21] attempt to resolve the issue by utilizing the terms *decision-oriented* and *conclusion-oriented* for categorization purposes, but then advise the reader that any semantic decision should be taken lightly since there are many borderline cases and crossovers within investigations. Reagan[23] offers over a dozen different definitions to demonstrate the ambiguity of the basic/applied dichotomy and states that these ambiguities can have a disruptive effect on the policy determinations in any field. Folta[24] concurs in stating that "the unfortunate labeling of pure versus applied and the subsequent implied conferral of prestige to one above the other frequently, and sometimes adversely affect the way research is conducted, problems are chosen, data analyzed, and the extent to which findings become of general significance."

It can be concluded from the foregoing that the crucial distinction between basic and applied research is not to be found in the source of the problem or in the methods used to conduct the exploration but in the purpose for which the investigation is carried out. In the case of theoretical research, the purpose is to solve a problem so as to test and expand knowledge, without regard to its later use. The nature of the research can be further characterized as cumulative and aimed at developing and testing a theoretical structure for the purpose of enhancing its explanatory power. Applied research aims to bring about change or to in some way influence the present state of operating properties in a situation.

This latter point seems to be very much a part of the many exhortations found in the nursing literature for more research that is clinically oriented and will make a difference in practice. Some of the criticism is, of course, more directly aimed at our former predilection for studying the nurse rather than the client. However, some believe that applied research produces a more immediate payoff for all concerned, by involving the practitioner in the research process and introducing findings that are of more immediate relevance to the improvement of clinical procedures. Insofar as the practitioners are concerned, it hardly seems reasonable to expect the majority to involve themselves directly in the conduct of research projects. Insofar as values are prime movers of behavior, Ackerman's observations appear closer to the mark:

> The crucial intervening variable between scientific theory and the quality of nursing practice appears to be the research attitude, rather than the research production of practitioners. In educational programs that prepare practitioners, then, the most important objective of research teaching must be the communication of an attitude of appreciation and enthusiasm for using research in the practice setting. Generating new knowledge is another matter, and for practitioners it may be extraneous.[25]

The argument about who should be carrying out research and what the features of the product should look like has at times reached feverish proportions. The statement has been made that nurses should eschew involving themselves in theorizing unless it can be shown that such activities make a difference in practice.[26] Before value judgments are made about what form of research is most closely allied to advancing the profession and its aims, there are several points that need to be kept in mind.

The notion that controlled investigation (and even this is a relative matter) of any phenomenon can yield definitive answers on a first trial denies the critical attributes of the statistical method of analysis and its cognitive significance. Much modern science, regardless of the specific goal of a study, is probabilistic in nature. The application of statical procedures implies that if a certain set of conditions exists, particular outcomes can be expected to occur with various degrees of certainty. This means that if *all* the elements that form the condition exist, the likelihood of recurrence of the dependent variable can be anticipated to a greater or lesser extent. The possibility that such circumstances can be duplicated in complex situations involving human beings is obviously close to zero. Nonetheless, with repeated experiments on similar and different groups, it is possible to demonstrate that the intervention in question remains likely to be effective even when background variables differ. It is also possible through assorted statistical maneuvers to eliminate certain elements, such as age, sex, or socioeconomic status, as influences on the results of the experiment.

The foregoing is not intended to discourage attempts to carry out research, but to make clear that there are simply too many variables that may contribute to chance findings to believe that there is a rapid scientific route to improving clinical practice. Neither basic nor applied research supplies quick or ready answers to problems that do not require replication and wary application. To believe otherwise is to deify research in a manner to which no hardheaded scientist would acquiesce. The argument that replication or refinement of a previous experiment stifles individual creativity does not hold water. Creativity in scientific endeavor is not primarily a matter of finding a novel problem but in designing inventive questions that will help to solve a problem and contribute working knowledge to a field.

Often the outcomes of applied research enjoy a far shorter life span than the outcomes which may at first appear too esoteric for day to day application. Ketefian[27] used the widely published outcomes of studies on techniques of temperature-taking as a focal point for illustrating that research findings are unknown and unheeded by the nursing community. The study has been cited rather widely in the nursing literature to demonstrate that research exerts little influence on clinical practice. However true this statement may be, it cannot be directly deduced from Ketefian's study. Such a conclusion ignores the fact that at the time of the survey electronic probes and a number of throw-away devices had been developed that were already on the market and in rather widespread use for estimating body temperature. We do not know how this may have influenced the respondents' answers, but it calls into question whether or not the temperature-taking studies were sufficiently germane to be considered seriously by clinicians. If this was indeed the case, a subject of technical importance in the late 1960s and early 1970s was of rapidly diminishing concern in less than five years.

The objective of this discussion of the limitations of applied research is not merely to exalt the stature of theoretical efforts. It is to highlight the need for a healthy balance between the two positions, which allows for diverse attacks on the solution and reconstruction of the definition of nursing and nursing practice. The purpose is also to prevent drawing the lines so narrowly around the definition of clinical practice that it becomes a synonym for application of technical procedures rather than a substantive means to deal with human problems from a nursing perspective. There is a clear difference between studying the most effective use of technology, and investigating the role of principles derived from nursing science in the solution of clinical problems. The meagre amount of nursing knowledge available for the latter purpose forms the primary argument for encouraging an all-out effort to develop theoretically oriented research. It is simply not possible to make use of what one does not have, and theoretical research provides a source point.

It is not uncommon to hear people say they are applying theory to practice. To make such a statement is to misunderstand the meaning of theory. A theory is no more than a set of speculative statements about the nature of some phenomenon. One makes use of the principles that are generated from systematically testing the theory. The theories of Sullivan, Freud, or Erickson can be used as a frame of reference for interpreting observable behavior, but this is not the same thing as applying knowledge about body mechanics to lifting a patient. The latter case utilizes principles derived from laws of physics as they relate to physiological functioning. To state that one method of lifting produces less strain than another is merely to classify the activity as a particular example of a more universal set of knowns and proceed accordingly. The former relies on inferences drawn from a theoretical stance that appear to "work" in practice. Failure to understand this difference has led more than a few to believe that much more verified knowledge about constructive intervention exists than is indeed the case. It also explains the fleeting popularity of certain schools of thought, among them schools involving the mother-child relationship, which are regularly replaced by "more contemporary views."

A BASIC/APPLIED RESEARCH CONTINUUM

Gage's *Handbook of Research on Teaching*[28] sets forth an interesting set of categories that describe a basic/applied continuum ranging from basic science through actual demonstration of methods. Although there is some overlap among the categories, it seems a helpful structure within which to visualize the research process. It does not oversimplify the route that must be taken to full application and makes clear that at any point a research product may need to be referred back either to the source of origin or to an even more elementary level for further clarification and scrutiny. It also provides an opportunity to demonstrate the numerous reasons why a single piece of research is too tenuous to move further along the continuum without additional supportive work.

Some minor alterations have been made in the original nomenclature that describes the system in order to facilitate its application to a nursing model rather than a pedagogical one. Some of the methodological problems, and strengths and weaknesses at each level, are suggested by research examples representing each category.

Entering the continuum from the basic science end, the categories are as follows:

1. Basic Science Content—Content Indifferent
2. Basic Science Content—Content Relevant

3. Investigation of Practically Oriented Nursing Problems
4. Experimentation on Problems of Practice in Controlled Situations
5. Clinical Trials
6. Dissemination of the Information Widely

Basic Science Content—
Content Indifferent

The context of research within this category is abstract and conceptual and is aimed at refining theory for the purpose of describing or predicting some phenomenon. Two studies by Newman,[29],[30] are examples of studies that fit into this category. Both studies are aimed at explaining the relation between motility and time estimation, with the second study attempting to eliminate a confounding variable created by subjects' attempts to compensate for the effect they thought variation in gait had on their estimation of elapsed time.

Obviously, to establish a link between body movement and an individual's estimation of the passage of time is an extremely complex task, which requires reduction of the overall goal to a point where some workable and circumscribed point of entry can be established. In order to accomplish this, Newman operationally defined mobility as rate of walking and time estimation as an individual's determination of how long a 40-second interval seemed to be. The necessity for control over the extraneous variables that are rampant in naturalistic settings placed further constraints on both the site of the investigations and the methodologies that might offer promise for shedding light on the nature of the relation between the variables.

Normal male subjects were tested while walking at different rates on a finely calibrated laboratory treadmill. In brief, the findings of the second study supported a linear relationship between time estimation and rate of walking and were consistent with the position taken by several theorists in the field. However, they did not entirely support the outcomes of the first study or indicate that the additional precautions taken to control subjects' compensatory behavior in estimating the passage of time were successful.

Newman suggests that one possibility for further study might be to investigate the relation between time estimation and motility among persons with actual disability that interferes with normal movement. However, proceeding in this direction may further confuse the *theoretical* relation by introducing a set of conditions which in themselves might be responsible for establishing a false connection. Thus the direction of choice would appear to be one that would contain future experiments within the Content—Indifferent category, through continued refinement of procedures aimed at teasing out the true relation between the study variables.

It may be argued that even if the relationship can be demonstrated, it is still not known whether or not generalizations can be made about people whose movement is restricted by disability. However, having clarified the theoretical position, it is then possible to move with more assurance along the science continuum to the second category, Basic Science Content—Content Relevant, to test the theory under new conditions. If the previously established relation fails to hold, then a search for confounding variables in the new situation can be systematically pursued.

Basic Science Content— Content Relevant

This category deals with studies that aim to define the knowledge necessary for practice, rather than studies on the needs of the practice situation per se. The need here is to develop systematic knowledge or to test theory at a conceptual rather than a practical level. Examples of this might be the studies of Foster,[31] Smith,[32] Barry,[33] and Capabianco[34] which examine the effect of personality variables and different auditory input on heart rate, motor activity, and time estimation while subjects are on bed rest.

The clinical relevance of these studies to practice is quite clear. However, considerable, thoughtful work needs to be done, before developing clinical experiments, to establish the specific interrelations that exist. The investigators narrowed their studies to a situation involving short-term bed rest (2.5 hours), during which time carefully screened subjects were exposed to three different types of auditory input. The three experimental situations utilized ambient sound, a series of intact radio tapes, and a series of the same tapes that had been segmented and randomly recombined within each episode.

An extensive group of hypotheses was formulated that, with the exception of two related to time estimation, failed to be supported by the data. This may have been due at least in part to unusual sensory experiences reported by subjects as having occurred during the period of bed rest.[35] These manifestations require further study at this level of investigation and/or at the level of practically oriented nursing problems. The original problem undertaken for study needs creative recasting in order to eliminate the influence of the undesired side effects, so that the critical theoretical links may be clearly established.

Doubt is often expressed about simulated environments and the constructions necessary to carry out such studies as are mentioned above, as to whether they correctly mirror the real world and consequently have valid implications for practice. Because these studies are designed to untangle theoretical puzzles, such questions are really premature unless an investigator presses the issue of their appropriateness for application. The most important question is whether or not the simulation is adequate to clarify the postulated theoretical stance.

Investigation of Practically Oriented Nursing Problems

The third classification, although not necessarily of a theory testing variety, still implies a theoretical rationale. Studies might take place in either a simulated environment or in an actual practice setting, as the following example illustrates.

Clinical observation led Errico[36] to become concerned about the procedures used in intensive care units to interpret to patients the events that occurred on cardiac monitors, which were clearly visible to them on the unit. She believed that the patients' understanding of these events was a significant factor in both their emotional and physical well-being. She used normal subjects who volunteered to be observed under three information conditions while on cardiac monitoring in an intensive care unit during periods when the patient census was low. She used blood pressure, heart rate, and respiration as indices of the dependent variable. Clear differences between treatment conditions were evident on the first two measurements. The ability of subjects to exert conscious control over breathing was questioned by the investigator as a component in its failure to discriminate among the various informational stimuli.

The degree to which either the volunteer character of this sample or the simulation, no matter how close an approximation to reality, is responsible for the outcome of the study cannot be determined without further examination and replication under similar conditions. Actual clinical experimentation before this is accomplished carries with it innumerable ethical dilemmas, to say nothing of the complications that are bound to ensue as the result of the various diagnoses, treatment regimens, and settings. It should also be clear that although a pragmatic relation may be established through either further laboratory work or clinical investigation, the *theoretical base* remains unexplored and obscure.

Experimentation on Problems of Practice in Controlled Situations

Studies of this kind ordinarily make use of practice situations in which real patients are the objects of study. Patients are carefully selected and whatever steps seem necessary are taken to bring environmental situations under control. This is admittedly a very difficult task which inevitably requires certain kinds of compromises. Many of these stem from the need to gain entry to sites that are willing to cooperate with the investigator or to find institutions that supply the required naturalistic settings. In so doing, it is often hard to determine what idiosyncratic variables may accompany these choices.

McGillicuddy's study[42] supplies an interesting case in point. She studied differences in behavior exhibited by children when they were hospitalized under rooming-in and non-rooming-in situations, as contrasted with non-hospitalized children. Because rooming-in is predominantly a system limited to private and semi-private accommodations, the sample was restricted in social class and drawn from three private voluntary hospitals. Non-hospitalized children were obtained from three private schools where parents with children in the required age group were asked to volunteer information.

The sample was limited to children between the ages of one and a half and four years of age who were hospitalized for more than one day but no more than ten days for acute disorders or minor surgery. The mothers of the children were administered a questionnaire at the time of the child's admission to the unit and one month after discharge.

The findings of the study indicate that children hospitalized with rooming-in did indeed show more movement toward mature behavior than the other two groups of children. This is seen as supporting the notions advanced by crisis theorists that stress situations may produce positive growth when the proper climate is provided. It may also be said that the mother's presence may allow a kind of environmental exploration and mastery that is not possible under other circumstances. It was also noted that children in the rooming-in group were the youngest of those in the sample and that the effect of this variable on the outcome remains obscure. This study could be profitably replicated in settings where random assignment to at least the rooming-in and non-rooming-in groups was possible, with the addition of suitable controls for managing the age variable.

Clinical Trials

At this point new ideas, approaches, or methods, which have been tested under controlled clinical situations such as the one described above, would be put into operation in representative settings. Systematic data would be collected to determine whether or not the typical nurse could apply the method appropriately and whether the response of patients would in general be a desirable one. Deviations from the expected outcome would be carefully noted in an effort to further refine the applicability of the method or to detect aspects of it that would indicate the need for further study before full acceptance.

Dissemination of the Information Widely

At last we come to the termination of the continuum. It is now that the necessary steps must be taken to insure the acceptance of the new approach and its uniform usage. These steps might include demonstrations, workshops, and seminars. The extent to which techniques advocated at this end of the continuum to promote practice innovations have actually been subjected to the scientific rigor of the preceding steps is often more questionable than the ordinary professional consumer realizes. Those who participate in such activities should have a sturdy belief in scientific methods and seek clarification on these points either through background reading or direct questioning of the presenter.

CONCLUSION

All those associated with nursing must learn to be discriminating and at the same time bold in their questioning of innovations derived from research. To be a consumer of research is not to be a passive tool of those who are actively pursuing knowledge. It is to provide essential information about the effect the knowledge that develops has on the course and outcome of pratice, and to identify the obstacles that remain.

There are no quick and easy solutions to nursing problems since they are, in the most intimate sense, the difficulties of people seeking decisions about how to attain a reasonable level of well-being under uncertain conditions. Rendering these decisions more predictable is the work of research in nursing.

REFERENCES

1. T.S. Kuhn, *International Encyclopedia of Unified Science. The Structure of Scientific Revolutions,* second edition, Vol. 2, No. 1 (Chicago: University of Chicago Press, 1970), p. 68.
2. American Nurses' Association, *Resolution on Priorities in Nursing Research,* submitted by the ANA Commission on Nursing Research before the House of Delegates at the 1974 Convention, June 12, 1974 and passed, *American Nurse* 6 (August 1974).
3. W.E. Deming, "The logic of evaluation," in E.L. Struening and M. Guttentag (eds.), *Handbook of Evaluation Research* Vol. 1 (Beverly Hills, Ca.: Sage, 1975), p. 53.
4. E.A. Suchman, *Evaluation Research* (New York: Russell Sage, 1967), pp. 61–62.

5. C. Weiss, "Evaluation research in the political context," in E.L. Struening and M. Guttentag (eds.), *Handbook of Evaluation Research* (Beverly Hills, Ca.: Sage, 1975), p. 13.

6. M.J. Zimmer, "Evaluation using patient health/wellness outcome criterion variables and standards," in *Issues in Evaluation Research* (Kansas City, Kan.: American Nurses' Association, 1976), p. 60.

7. M.J. Goran, *et al.,* "The PSRO hospital review system," *Medical Care* 13 (April 1975): 17.

8. H. Yura and M. Walsh, *The Nursing Process,* second edition (New York: Appleton, 1973), p. 14.

9. D.E. Johnson, "Development of theory: A requisite for nursing as a primary health profession," *Nurs Res* 23 (September–October 1974): 373.

10. L. Sharp, "The behavioral scientist in nursing research," *Nurs Res* 13 (Fall 1964): 330.

11. K. Andreoli and C.E. Thompson, "The nature of science in nursing," *Image* 9 (June 1977): 32–37.

12. D.E. Johnson, "The nature of a science of nursing," *Nurs Outlook* 7 (May 1959): 291–94.

13. M.E. Rogers, *An Introduction to the Theoretical Basis of Nursing* (Philadelphia: Davis, 1970).

14. S.R. Gortner, "Research for a Practice Profession," *Nurs Res* 24: 3, May–June 1975, pp. 193–96.

15. A. Jacox, "Research in nursing–a contemporary view," *American Nurse* (September 15, 1976): 4–5.

16. D. Diers, "This I believe . . . about nursing research," *Nurs Outlook* 18 (November 1970): 50–54.

17. G. Holton, "Scientific optimism and societal concerns," *Hastings Cent. Rep.* 5 (December 1975): 39.

18. J.S. Brunner, *Beyond the Information Given* (New York: Norton, 1973), p. 145.

19. D.E. Crowley, "Perspectives of pure science," *Nurs Res* 17 (November–December 1968): 497–98.

20. G.K. Bixler, "What is research?" *Nurs Res* 1 (June 1952): 7.

21. L.J. Cronbach and P. Suppes (eds.), *Research for Tomorrow's Schools,* Report of the Committee on Educational Research of the National Academy of Education (London: Macmillan, 1969), pp. 19–20.

22. New York Telephone, "New material made at Bell Labs," *Weekly Summary for Management* (September 23, 1976).

23. M. Reagan, "Basic and applied research: A meaningful distinction?" *Science* 155 (March 1967): 1383–86.

24. J. Folta, "Perspectives of an applied scientist," *Nurs Res* 17 (November–December 1968): 502.

25. W. Ackerman, "The place of research in the master's program," *Nurs Outlook* 24 (December 1976): 754–58.

26. J. Dickoff and P. James, "Clarity to what end?" (commentary on Walker's "Toward a clearer understanding of the concept of nursing theory"), *Nurs Res* 20 (November–December 1971): 501.

27. S. Ketefian, "Application of selected nursing research findings into nursing practice: A pilot study," *Nurs Res* 24 (March–April 1975): 89–92.
28. N.L. Gage, "Paradigms for research on teaching," in N.L. Gage (ed.), *Handbook of Research on Teaching* (Chicago: Rand McNally, 1963), pp. 97–98.
29. M.A. Newman, "Time estimation in relation to gait tempo," *Percept. Mot. Skills* 34 (April 1972): 359–66.
30. M.A. Newman, "Movement tempo and the experience of time," *Nurs Res* 25 (July–August 1976): 273–79.
31. C. Foster, "The relation between internal-external control, environmental auditory input and gross motor activity in bed confined individuals," unpublished doctoral dissertation (New York University, 1974).
32. M.J. Smith, "An investigation of changes in judgment of duration with different patterns of auditory information for individuals confined to bed," unpublished doctoral dissertation (New York University, 1974).
33. M.J. Barry, "The relation between introversion-extraversion, auditory input, and motor activity in bed confined individuals," unpublished doctoral dissertation (New York University, 1974).
34. A. Capabianco, "An investigation of the relationship between auditory environments and pulse rate changes in bed-confined young adults," unpublished doctoral dissertation (New York University, 1975).
35. F. Downs, "Bed rest and sensory disturbances," *Am. J. Nurs.* 75 (March 1974): 434–38.
36. E. Errico, "Investigation of the relationship between cardiac monitoring and information feedback and blood pressure, heart rate and respiration," unpublished doctoral dissertation (New York University, 1975).
37. M. McGillicuddy, "A study of the relationship between mothers' rooming-in during their children's hospitalization and changes in selected areas of children's behavior," in F. Downs and M.A. Newman (eds.), *A Sourcebook of Nursing Research* (Philadelphia: Davis, 1977), pp. 64–67.

CHAPTER FIVE

THE NATURE AND DEVELOPMENT OF CONCEPTUAL FRAMEWORKS

Carolyn A. Williams

Identification of a conceptual framework has become a sine qua non for educators responsible for programs of nursing education (particularly baccalaureate programs), and for those seeking funding for research undertakings. Master's or doctoral students seeking faculty approval to move ahead with research projects are also frequently aware of the necessity of presenting conceptual frameworks. Despite tacit acknowledgement that conceptual frameworks are essential to successful reviews by accrediting bodies, review committees, and faculty, considerable confusion surrounds such questions as:

What constitutes a conceptual framework?
What substantive purposes do conceptual frameworks serve?
How are they identified and refined?

These questions will be addressed here. Also, it will be argued that while we are always operating to some extent within conceptual frameworks, there are variations in the degree to which we are aware of them, and in their specificity.

Following introductory terminological comments, the importance of explicit conceptual frameworks to the development of research and to thoughtful decision making in patient care will be discussed. Finally, selected issues pertinent to developing useful conceptual frameworks will be considered.

BACKGROUND

For nursing researchers and educators the last decade and a half has been a period in which much interest has been generated in developing a scientific basis for nursing practice.[1,2,3] It is frequently argued that research is the only route to developing such a knowledge base. But at the same time, nurse researchers are often frustrated by an awareness that many nursing administrators and nursing clinicians place little value on the research process and make little use of the results of research in their decision making. The reader may ask, "What has the above dilemma to do with conceptual frameworks?" The answer is: a very great deal.

With the growing interest in patient care research there has arisen an eagerness to determine whether nursing care makes a difference. In the primary care field, for example, this interest has been channeled into attempts designed to assess the impact of nurse practitioners on patient outcomes and organizational outcomes.[4,5,6]

Parallel to the growing interest in nursing research, there has been considerable dialogue on the issue of theory development in nursing.[7-10] Two kinds of literature have developed: one deals with the process of theory development and another consists of attempts to actually develop what some refer to as theories of nursing.[11-13] The nature of the relationship between theory development, research, and practice is an issue particularly germane to our discussion. To place the discussion in a clinical perspective, we suggest that from the point of view of the thoughtful clinician who is attempting to determine how she can most effectively intervene with patients who have certain characteristics in common (e.g., newly diagnosed hypertensives who are otherwise asymptomatic) to facilitate a desired outcome (achievement of normotensive status), the vision of the ideal knowledge base is congruent with the vision of the researcher-theorist seriously interested in theory development. The clinician needs a basis for action, one which will predictably accomplish the desired objective. The researcher-theorist's ultimate goal is to develop a theory, which as defined by Kerlinger is: ". . . a set of interrelated constructs (concepts), definitions, and propositions that present a systematic view of phenomena by specifying relations among variables, with the purpose of explaining and predicting the phenomena."[14] Thus, if the clinician has access to—and uses as a basis for dealing with such patients—the knowledge generated from studies which led to development of tested theory for facilitating given patient responses, her practice will probably be more effective and may be considered scientific.

Clearly, for a practice discipline the ideal (and the priority) is to develop practice theories which will guide clinicians in what should be assessed in patients and what interventions might be most productive. This is the goal toward which many are working who are interested in developing scientifically-derived knowledge as a basis for clinical nursing practice. The practical importance of theory in guiding clinical decisions is in itself sufficient reason for becoming more familiar with the relevant terminology, as a first step toward contributing meaningfully to actual theory development.

THEORETICAL TERMINOLOGY

As background for further discussion of the relationship between research, theory, and practice, it is useful to consider terminology basic to discussions of theory development in all fields. Clarification of the following terms is particularly important: concept, variable, hypothesis, conceptual or theoretical framework, theory, and model.

Concepts, Hypotheses, Theories

The term *concept* is fundamental to any discussion of theory. As used by philosophers of science and many researchers, the term refers to a category or class of objects or phenomena. In other words, concepts represent an abstract way of referring to the real world. Examples of familiar concepts which refer to clearly visible entities in the world are: dog, cat, house, patient, family, and nurse practitioner. Concepts which refer to phenomena not directly observable are usually referred to as constructs. Examples include: intelligence, ego, and age. Concepts which can take on more than one value are called variables. As distinguished from concepts, hypotheses or propositions are statements which specify the relationship between two or more concepts. For example, "preoperative teaching is negatively associated with length of hospital stay" is a proposition (hypothesis) which specifies a relationship between the concepts (variables).

Before leaving the topic of concepts, it might be useful to point out two types of statements which are frequently called concepts but which, according to the above terminology, are propositions. The first is simply an hypothesis, e.g., "In order for a nursing plan to be effective the patient must be involved." The second is a statement of objectives, e.g., "The primary goal is to maintain the patient's optimum physical and psychosocial functioning." Each example involves several concepts: nursing plan, patient, goal, and functioning. In the first example, an hypothesis, the positive relationship between nursing plan effectiveness and patient involvement is stated. The second statement is a simple objective involving two concepts—physical functioning and psychosocial functioning. Although those statements may represent a popular understanding of the term concept, such use is confusing and not consistent with the prevalent usage in research literature. Perhaps it is the frequent labeling of such phrases as concepts in undergraduate nursing programs which is responsible in part for the difficulty which so many nurses have in understanding the usual scientific use of the term concept. In discussing concepts as classes or categories, and concepts as statements (propositions, hypotheses), Scheffler, a philosopher, had the following comment:

> Putting the matter in terms of categories and simplifying, we may express the point as follows: conceptualization relates both to the idea of categories for the sorting of items and to the idea of expectation, belief, or hypothesis . . . it links up with the notion of *category* [concept] and, also, with the quite different notion of *hypothesis*. The very same category system, surely, is compatible with alternative, and indeed conflicting hypotheses.[15]

As previously noted, a theory as defined by most philosophers has certain attributes: the concepts are clearly defined, there are propositions or hypotheses which relate the concepts, these propositions are themselves systematically interrelated, and the propositions are empirically testable. We have used the terms proposition and hypothesis interchangeably, which may be sufficient for our purposes; however, in well-developed fields such as physics some propositions which have not been refuted by repeated empirical testing, and are thus considered to be well supported, are referred to as laws (e.g., Boyle's Law: "The pressure of a gas at constant temperature is inversely proportional to its volume."). Those more tentative propositions are called hypotheses. An additional point frequently made in distinguishing well developed theories from isolated hypotheses is that theories possess general propositions sometimes referred to as axioms, postulates, or premises from which more specific theorems or hypotheses are deduced. For example, Brodbeck defines a theory as "a deductively connected set of laws. Some of these laws, the axioms or postulates of the theory, logically imply others, the theorems."[16] The state of the art is such that it is only in the more formalized physical and biological sciences that such well developed theories or the theoretical ideal is approached. In discussing this point Jacox quotes a comment by Blalock, a sociologist: "For a considerable period of time, social scientists will have to settle for highly tentative theories based on axioms that are really nothing more than rather plausible assumptions."[17]

Conceptual/Theoretical Frameworks

Are theories and conceptual frameworks distinguishable? Recognizing that within the literature there is considerable and somewhat confusing overlap in the use of terms such as theory, conceptual framework, theoretical framework, and model, we will make distinctions for the purpose of our discussion. First, if we define a conceptual framework as a group of concepts plus a set of propositions which spell out the relationships between those concepts, then all theories by definition are conceptual frameworks. However, not all conceptual frameworks meet the criteria of a theory as previously discussed, and thus cannot be considered theories because in many cases the concepts are not sufficiently well defined to allow for empirical testing of hypotheses. Here it might be useful to suggest that most of what are referred to as theories in nursing are better viewed as conceptual frameworks. These vary in (1) the degree to which concepts are specified and can be measured and (2) the extent to which relationships among the concepts are made explicit and are suitable for empirical testing. Thus, a conceptual framework may be usefully understood as a set of concepts and, in addition, a group of statements which spell out how the concepts are interrelated.

The term *framework* suggests something which is incomplete but which provides broad outlines and which can be filled in or filled out in order to produce a more complete structure. The distinction between a theory and a conceptual framework, admittedly somewhat fuzzy, appears then to be a matter of the range of phenomena included and the degree of specificity of the concepts and hypotheses. Conceptual frameworks are broader, more general, and more vague. They are not easily submitted to empirical testing. Theories, by contrast, tend to deal with more limited phenomena, to be more precise (even to the point of including quantifiable relationships), and to have their concepts sufficiently well defined to allow for empirical testing. By these criteria Roy's work[13,18] is clearly an example of a conceptual framework rather than a theory; adaptation is very broad and needs much more clarification and definition of terms before it will allow for measurement and test. Although the terms theoretical framework and conceptual framework are sometimes used interchangeably, we tend to prefer conceptual framework as a more general term which does not imply that formal relationships are specified among the concepts.

Models

The term "model" is used with several common but different meanings. (1) Sometimes it is used simply as a synonym for "theory."[19] (2) Sometimes it is a synonym for "conceptual framework" (as in the Roy adaptation model/ conceptual framework). (3) Sometimes "model" is used in place of "theory" by way of emphasizing the tentative and merely suggestive nature of what is being said. (4) Sometimes a theory which is quantified to the extent that it, or parts of it, can be expressed mathematically in equations is called a model (a "mathematical model"). That is, hypotheses of the theory state that certain mathematical relationships exist between the variables, and such relationships are expressible in equations (e.g., multiple regression equations).[20] (5) Sometimes "model" is used to refer to one area of knowledge which, it is hoped, will display useful analogies with another and less well-known area. The model can then be used as a source of ideas—a means of suggesting further investigations, of generating hypotheses. For example, in this sense a computer is often used as a model for the human brain.*[21] A good deal more is known about how computers work than is known about how the brain works, so computer structure is used as a source of hypotheses about brain structure. Computers have central processing units, core memory units, and long-term storage units—using the computer as a model for the brain suggests the hypothesis that there are three similarly distinguishable "units" in the brain.

USING CONCEPTUAL FRAMEWORKS

Once we acknowledge that theory is valuable as a basis for action and that formal theories for those concerned, at least in part, with behavioral issues (as are nurses) are yet to be developed, the importance of conceptual frameworks as a stage in theory development becomes evident. Rather than waste energy lamenting our lack of formal theories, it may be more fruitful to consider seriously where we are, what we do have and how we can encourage its

---

*For those interested in further discussion regarding models, Brodbeck's paper[16] describes several other technical senses in which the term "model" is used in science.

refinement. Therefore, much of the remaining discussion will explore topics pertinent to an understanding of conceptual frameworks, their usefulness, and strategies for making them explicit.

Conceptual frameworks serve the basic purpose of providing focus—this can be at the level of a discipline, of a curriculum, or of a particular investigation. One way of viewing the work of nurses such as Orem[12] and Roy,[13,18] whose efforts are sometimes referred to as attempts to develop a theory of nursing, is to suggest that rather than develop theory in the sense in which we have defined it, their contribution has been to help clarify the focus of nursing as a discipline through the explication of conceptual frameworks. Indeed, this general intention seems clear in the preface of Orem's book, *Nursing: Concepts of Practice.*

> The book is not a substitute for nor does it stand in opposition to other works in the developing nursing literature. By providing a structured framework of nursing in relevant concepts and principles . . . the book affords position and meaning to other expositions of nursing and to the developing body of knowledge about the nursing process and the technologies of nursing.[22]

Questions about how nursing is defined and how it is differentiated from other disciplines are frequently pondered by nurses, graduate students in nursing, and some segments of the public. Since disciplines are usually defined or differentiated from others by their concepts, their hypotheses, and the questions to which they seek answers, the contribution of those who seek to develop such conceptual frameworks is considerable.

Many readers have had exposure to a conceptual framework from participation in a nursing curriculum either as a student or faculty member. In view of this general familiarity, it may be useful to comment on the development and use of frameworks for curriculum purposes in order to relate these to the development of a framework for a particular investigation or series of investigations.

The value of a conceptual framework at the curriculum level is acknowledged by inclusion in the National League for Nursing's *Revised Draft of Criteria for Appraisal of Baccalaureate and Higher Degree Programs in Nursing.* The criteria statement is as follows: "The curriculum implements the philosophy, purposes, and objectives of the program(s) and is developed within a conceptual framework."[23] This definition of conceptual framework is provided: "Conceptual framework is a distinct, systematic organization of concepts which stems from the philosophy and purposes and gives direction to the curriculum."[24] In arguing for the value of a conceptual framework, both Harms[25] and Gordon[26] comment on its role in guiding decisions about curriculum content. More specifically, Gordon has illustrated how crucial concepts can be identified (she used three—adaptation, client systems, and preventive intervention), showed diagrammatically how the concepts might interact, and suggested the manner in which organization of the curriculum could be derived from the framework. Other accounts in recent nursing literature describe the use of Maslow's hierarchy of need[27] and Roy's adaptation model[28] as the conceptual basis for curricula.

Conceptual frameworks identified for either a curriculum or a study have the same basic purpose of focusing, ruling some things in as relevant, and ruling others out due to their lesser importance. However, conceptual frameworks for particular studies differ from those utilized in curriculum development in significant ways. The first is the specificity with which the concepts are defined. For the most part, concepts used in curricular frameworks are somewhat vague, or not sufficiently defined to admit measurement, whereas in the context of a particular investigation it is essential that the concepts be clearly defined and indicators selected or developed for their measurement. An illustration of this distinction is provided by an account documenting the efforts of five graduate students to use a conceptual framework—Roy's adaptation model—as a basis for patient assessment.[29] The generality of Roy's four adaptive modes or concepts (basic physiological needs, self-concept, role function, and interdependence) may be acceptable for use in focusing or structuring a curriculum, and her model has successfully served as a framework for curricula. However, the students who wanted to assess individual patients in a systematic manner were faced with the need to agree on how the concepts would be specifically defined and empirically identified in their project. An assessment tool was devised but the report states, ". . . some difficulty was encountered in trying to determine to which mode some of the items in the assessment tool referred. Increasingly, the students realized that some aspects of the self-concept, role function, and interdependence modes appeared to overlap."[30] Thus, the need to be specific about definitions for the purpose of a particular project pointed out the need for further refinement of the concepts. Acknowledging this need, the author of the model commented as follows.

In regard to the difficulties that the graduate students encountered in testing the model, I recognize the problems involved in the overlap among the adaptive modes. This had always been a problem. Nevertheless, I am still intuitively convinced that there is some unique content related to each one which has implications for interventions, and I therefore continue to keep them all. However, only practice and research related to the problem areas and their interventions can demonstrate whether or not this is the best way of systematically assessing the adaptive person. In the meantime, I can only sympathize with the practical difficulties involved in distinguishing behaviors by modes. I would encourage practitioners who discover meaningful delineations to communicate these to me directly or through publication.[31]

Although it may be obvious to many readers, there is some value in pointing to a second distinction between the conceptual framework as used in studies and as used in curricula: namely, the objective of a study is usually either (1) to describe phenomena by categorizing and enumerating them, (2) to answer specific questions concerning the relationships between two or more concepts (variables), or (3) to submit to test hypothesized relationships between concepts. In contrast, the relationships between concepts in curricula are considered at a more general level and are either assumed to exist or have been found to exist through empirical testing. The Roy model, as described by its originator in the following phrase, seems to be at the stage of assumption.

While the model did grow out of my experience as a nurse, it is primarily a deductive model [derived from theory in other fields]. It has not yet been submitted to the rigors of clinical research that will be necessary to establish its validity. The few small pilot studies that have been done in no way approach the extensive, systematic program of research that I believe is needed in the future.[31]

DEVELOPING CONCEPTUAL FRAMEWORKS

Implicit and Explicit Conceptual Frameworks

To some extent everyone already has a conceptual framework, in that we all have assumptions and presuppositions about how the world is put together, and we already have a set of concepts which we use for categorizing things in our experience. For example, we all operate with the concepts of space, time, sameness, difference, and physical object; and we all share a certain belief

which expresses relationships among those concepts, viz., that different physical objects cannot be in the same place at the same time. In the clinical situation different practitioners have different ways of approaching the same
patients, and in so doing some providers consider certain information more
relevant than do other providers. What is popularly referred to as the medical
model suggests a general view of patients which many physicians share and
indicates the type of data they consider most relevant. Other professionals,
particularly nurses, feel the need for alternative viewpoints—hence the efforts
of individuals such as Orem,[12] Roy,[13] and more recently Jacox.[10]

Whether they are explicit or not, the conceptual frameworks within which
we operate have a major role in suggesting what is important to study. This
point is clearly made by Hempel in his argument against what some view as
the four stages in an ideal approach to scientific inquiry: "(1) observation and
recording of all facts; (2) analysis and classification of these facts; (3) inductive derivation of generalizations from them; and (4) further testing of the
generalizations."[32] Hempel's first criticism of this approach to inquiry, which
he terms as the "narrow inductivist conception of scientific inquiry," is as
follows:

> First, a scientific investigation as here envisaged could never be carried
> out, for a collection of all the facts would have to await the end of the
> world, so to speak; and even all the facts up to now cannot be col-
> lected, since there are an infinite number and variety of them. Are we
> to examine, for example, all the grains of sand in all the deserts and on
> all the beaches, and are we to record their shapes, their weights, their
> chemical composition, their distances from each other, their constantly
> changing temperature, and their equally changing distance from the
> center of the moon? Are we to record the floating thoughts that cross
> our minds in the tedious process? The shapes of the clouds overhead,
> the changing color of the sky? The construction and the trade name of
> our writing equipment? Our own life histories and those of our fellow
> investigators? All these, and untold other things, are, after all, among
> "all the facts up to now."
>
> Perhaps, then, all that should be required in the first phase is that all
> the relevant facts be collected. But relevant to what?[33]

Hempel goes on to say that ". . . what particular sorts of data it is reasonable
to collect is not determined by the problem under study, but by a tentative
answer to it that the investigator entertains in the form of a conjecture or
hypothesis."[34] He further comments:

In sum, the maxim that data should be gathered without guidance by antecedent hypotheses about the connections among the facts under study is self-defeating, and it is certainly not followed in scientific inquiry. On the contrary, tentative hypotheses are needed to give direction to a scientific investigation. Such hypotheses determine, among other things, what data should be collected at a given point in a scientific investigation.[35]

A second criticism Hempel makes of the narrow inductivist approach is that tentative hypotheses are necessary in order to clarify and analyze the data in a meaningful manner.[35] The relevance of these points is that they increase our awareness of the fact that what we study and how we go about it are influenced by a conceptual framework. There is no pure, completely unbiased collection of data. Thus, unless we make our conceptual framework explicit, we are operating on implicit, unexamined assumptions and hypotheses. And if we remain in this state our efforts may be disappointing.

At the beginning of a study the process of developing an explicit conceptual framework is helpful in clarifying our thinking, suggesting variables and relationships which should be considered in our design. It provides for the integration of otherwise scattered and unrelated bits of information; that is, it provides coherence and organization. At the stage of data analysis the conceptual framework aids in interpretation by suggesting what the ramifications of particular findings might be. Finally, the conceptual framework aids in figuring out "where to go next." These are clearly arguments in favor of developing conceptual frameworks, but how does one go about the practical task of doing so? Although there is no one way to develop a conceptual framework, some general comments about the process may be useful.

Ideally, research in nursing practice should be related to clinical problems and should provide answers to questions which will influence practitioners' decisions. Thus, one might see a problem such as a high rate of medication errors in ambulatory, chronically ill patients and seek data which would provide a basis for dealing with the problem. However, to move ahead with the investigation one must have some general notions (tentative hypotheses) about why these patients are having so much trouble. Possibilities might include lack of patient teaching, lack of patient interest and motivation, a medication plan made without patient participation and not compatible with the patient's daily schedule, too many medications, etc. Depending on the investigator's conceptual framework, one or some combination of the above, or an unmentioned possibility, would be selected for study. The ensuing study—which might be limited to a descriptive account of the situation, or might extend to attempting an intervention based on some hypotheses regarding factors associated with the problem—could possibly proceed with no formal, explicit attention given to the conceptual framework. Of course, definitions of the variables would have to be developed and methods devised for measuring them—the finished study might result in statistically and clinically useful associations between variables of interest. Yet, some might comment that although it was empirically interesting the study lacked theoretical importance. Would that be a significant criticism?

From the preceding comments by Hempel it should be clear that the study did not develop in a conceptual vacuum. The basic limitation, however, may be that since the implicit conceptual framework was not made explicit and was not scrutinized or examined in relationship to alternatives, important variables or hypotheses were not considered and thus clear decisions were not made as to whether the study design should or should not include them. Here it is important to distinguish between (a) simply making implicit conceptual frameworks explicit and (b) the process involved in developing a well thought out, integrative conceptual framework. The latter involves taking the beginning explicit framework and scrutinizing it through comparison with the ways others look at the phenomena of interest (involving a thorough literature review and including the identification of frameworks and theories from other fields); probably adapting it in the process of refinement; perhaps discarding it and adopting another in light of what one finds in the literature; or inventing a new framework. These comments may seem to apply only to those whose study arises from a practical clinical situation. Yet even in cases where one is attempting deductively to move from theory in one field to test situations in nursing practice (as did Johnson in part, discussion to follow), the value of examining alternative frameworks and relating several cannot be underestimated. This is particularly so in many nursing practice studies which are complex due to the fact that interest is not limited to understanding relationships among patient characteristics but extends to the question of how provider participation will influence these relationships and, especially, how certain desired outcomes can be achieved (i.e., developing situation-producing theory).[9,36]

A second limitation imposed by the absence of a clear conceptual framework is that the investigator may be hampered in the interpretative phase by lack of awareness of the full scope of the study's implications. An additional limitation is that the contribution of the study may not be recognized for what it is. For example, unbeknown to the investigator the study might have generated information which either supported or refuted hypotheses held by others, particularly researchers in more basic fields. Thus, the study may fail to contribute maximally to the development of an organized body of knowledge.

Within the nursing literature there are examples of studies in which the conceptual frameworks are not explicitly presented; there are fewer examples, it seems, in which they have been. By way of illustrating some of the preceding remarks it may be useful to comment briefly on the contrast between two sets of studies in recent nursing literature. The first, by Lindeman and Van Aernam,[37,38] examines the effects of two different approaches to preoperative teaching on patient ability to cough and deep breathe, on average length of hospital stay, and on the use of postoperative analgesics. The second set, by Johnson and colleagues,[39-41] deals with the effects of the structuring of patients' expectations on their reactions to threatening events. Both groups of investigations have definite clinical relevance in that they provide data which are useful in decision making, and both have been highly influential in stimulating other investigators. In the first set, the value of preoperative teaching is clearly supported; and in the second, information about the sensations which accompany certain procedures is found to be useful in reducing patient distress. However, the studies differ considerably in the extent to which the conceptual framework is made explicit and explained.

Although there is a brief literature review in the Lindeman studies, no explicit comments are offered concerning a conceptual framework. On the other hand, in each of the papers by Johnson and associates there is considerable discussion regarding the theoretical underpinnings for the investigation. It is difficult to say which set of studies will be the more influential in actually improving clinical practice. Nonetheless, the presence of an explicitly considered conceptual framework in the Johnson studies aids the reader in thinking of other kinds of circumstances in which the hypothesized relationship might be expected to hold. That is to say, Johnson's basic hypothesis—"discrepancy between expectations about sensations and experience during a threatening event results in distress"[42]—which is explicitly developed in the context of recent work in psychology, is more obviously generalizable than is Lindeman's—"structured preoperative teaching would significantly increase the adult surgical patient's ability to cough and deep breathe. . . ."[43] Although Johnson is quite specific about the nature of the information concerning sensations which is to be communicated to patients, her hypothesis, by virtue of being embedded in a broader conceptual framework, more readily suggests other possible applications in different kinds of clinical situations. It is not difficult to think of a number of clinical circumstances in which patients are experiencing threatening events and in which the hypothesized relationship can be expected to hold. Although there may also be many clinical circumstances in which patients could be profitably taught such skills as coughing and deep breathing, Lindeman's hypothesis, which is specific to pre-surgical patients, is not as obviously generalizable to other patient groups.

Toward Theory

In the introductory remarks it was suggested that the ideal outcome of the research process is to develop practice theories which hold up under empirical test and can then be used to guide clinicians in assessing patients and predicting what interventions might be most productive. Further, it was argued that as a field nursing is at the conceptual framework stage of theory development.

In order to develop well-specified theories, it will be necessary to designate concepts more clearly and in measurable terms and, most importantly, to make explicit the hypothesized relationships between the concepts. At this point it may be useful to comment briefly on approaches to hypothesis generation—deciding which concepts are related under specified conditions. One approach is to start with premises from nursing or another field and deduce an hypothesis relevant to nursing practice. Deduction is often viewed as a form of reasoning in which a less general conclusion or hypothesis is logically derived from more general premises, either untested and assumed to be true or empirically tested and unrefuted. The conclusion, an hypothesis, can be empirically tested in an investigation and if refuted (not supported by the data), the deduced hypothesis and at least one of the premises are considered false.

Broadly speaking, Johnson's work is an example of such an approach, although we suggest her efforts were not deductive in a pure sense. In describing the process used in developing the hypothesis that "discrepancy between expectations about sensations and experience during a threatening event results in distress,"[42] Johnson pointed to a series of what she referred to as assumptions from the psychological literature. As she detailed them, these assumptions were: "stimuli are received and processed to extract the information that they contain, . . . thought processes are involved in attitudes and emotions as well as behaviors that guide performance, [and] . . . the processes guiding evaluation and performance require different information and are independent of each other. . . ."[42] According to Johnson these assumptions were used to examine patients' experiences during threatening events. And in doing so she noted that the reports of patients suggested they had "sought information from which to form expectations about the impending events and they compared expectations with the experience."[42] Johnson then reasoned that these observations could be explained by the following general hypothesis from the psychology literature: "discrepancy between expectations and experience results in an unpleasant emotion, and the more discrepant the expectations and experience, the greater the unpleasantness. . . ."[42] However, she recognized that this hypothesis was too general to be useful in guiding nursing action, since patient care situations are complex and there are many opportunities for discrepancies between experience and expectations. Therefore, she found it necessary to specify the type of discrepancies which would be related to negative outcomes. As Johnson described it, her hypothesis that a discrepancy between expectations about physical sensations and experience might be productive of distress emerged from her examination of data from laboratory and clinical studies which dealt with threatening events. The following statement summarizes in Johnson's words the overall process which led to the development of her basic hypothesis and guided her program of research.

> Beginning with four assumptions from psychology and building on observations from nursing practice, the laboratory, and clinical studies, I arrived at a hypothesis about the processes underlying distress during threatening events. This allowed me to predict one of the conditions that will increase or decrease distress. Specifically, accurate expectations about the physical sensations a subject is to experience will reduce distress during the confrontation with a threatening event.[44]

It seems clear that Johnson's specific hypothesis was in part suggested by theoretical formulations in psychology (which she called general assumptions) and in that sense could be considered deductive. Yet her move from (a) the general hypothesis regarding a discrepancy in expectations and experiences and unpleasant emotion to (b) the specific hypothesis concerning the relationship of distress to the discrepancy between expectation about physical sensations and experience could be viewed as an example of induction. Her comments imply that she came upon that particular hypothesis through looking at laboratory and clinical data. In other words, the hypothesis was not deduced directly from the propositions in psychology but was, in part, induced from observations which were admittedly focused as a function of the assumptions with which she was working. However, it is conceivable that another hypothesis could have been induced from the same observations.

In contrast to deduction, induction is often thought of as reasoning in which one begins with less general premises (frequently reported observations) and uses these as a basis for arriving at a more general hypothesis. Further, the link between the data and the conclusion is not a necessary one. The following comments by Hempel are helpful in clarifying the nature of an inductive approach to hypothesis generation.

> There are, then, no generally applicable "rules of induction," by which hypotheses or theories can be mechanically derived or inferred from

empirical data. The transition from data to theory requires creative imagination. Scientific hypotheses and theories are not derived from observed facts, but invented in order to account for them. They constitute guesses at the connections that might obtain between the phenomena under study, at uniformities and patterns that might underlie their occurrence. "Happy guesses" of this kind require great ingenuity, especially if they involve a radical departure from current modes of scientific thinking, as did, for example, the theory of relativity and quantum theory.[45]

To summarize, both inductive and deductive reasoning can be utilized in arriving at hypotheses. It is not an either/or situation. In fact, some of the more heuristic and clinically productive research may be based on hypotheses which resulted—as did Johnson's—from a combination of deductive and inductive reasoning. Awareness of this is useful in considering the enterprise of theory development in nursing, since it gives attention to the complementary role of theory in other disciplines and to clinically relevant observations made by nurse clinicians involved in rendering service.

If the process of hypothesis generation begins with theory from another field and proceeds in a deductive manner, it would be advisable, prior to initiating a study, to give attention to the clinical viability of the hypothesis. Such consideration may identify conditions (variables) which would influence the hypothesized relationships or, through an inferential process, lead to a new hypothesis. On the other hand, development of the hypothesis may be initiated from inferences based on clinical observations. In this case, it would be advantageous to make the assumptions explicit and to consider how the hypothesis under consideration compares with the way others look at the phenomena of interest. This would include considering conceptual frameworks and theories from other fields and on occasion modifying the original hypothesis in light of them. Regardless of the starting point, success in theory development will be enhanced through the active participation of clinicians who are thoroughly familiar with the practice arena, and with current theories and data in the field.

REFERENCES

1. R. Schlotfeld, "Research in Nursing and Research Training for Nurses: Retrospect and Prospect," *Nurs Res* 24 (May–June 1975): 177–83.
2. S. Gortner, "Research for a Practice Profession," *Nurs Res* 24 (May–June 1975) 193–97.

3. D. Bloch, "Evaluation of Nursing Care in Terms of Process and Outcome," *Nurs Res* 24 (July–August 1975): 256–63.
4. C. Lewis and B. Resnik, "Nurse Clinics and Progressive Ambulatory Patient Care," *N. Engl. J. Med.* 277 (March 20, 1969): 645–49.
5. D. Sackett, W. Spitzer, M. Gent, and R. Roberts, "The Burlington Randomized Trial of the Nurse Practitioner: Health Outcomes of Patients," *Ann. Intern. Med.* 80 (February 1974): 137–42.
6. S. Henshaw, "Evaluation of Nurse Practitioners in a General Medical Clinic," in S. Henshaw (ed.), *Three Studies of the Acceptance and Impact of Nurse Practitioners* (New York: Cornell University, New York Hospital School of Nursing, Division of Continuing Education, 1976).
7. J. Berthold, "Prologue to Symposium on Theory Development in Nursing," *Nurs Res* 17 (May–June 1968): 196–97.
8. J. Dickoff and P. James, "Researching Research's Role in Theory Development," *Nurs Res* 17 (May–June 1968): 204–6.
9. J. Dickoff, P. James, and E. Wiedenback, "Theory in a Practice Discipline: Part I, Practice Oriented Theory," *Nurs Res* 17 (September–October 1968): 415–35.
10. A. Jacox, "Theory Construction in Nursing: an Overview," *Nurs Res* 23 (January–February 1974):4–13.
11. D. Johnson, "Nature of a Science of Nursing," *Nurs Res* 7 (May 1959): 291–94.
12. D. Orem, *Nursing: Concepts of Practice* (New York: McGraw-Hill, 1971).
13. S.C. Roy, "Adaptation: a Conceptual Framework for Nursing," *Nurs Outlook* 18 (March 1970): 42–45.
14. F. Kerlinger, *Foundations of Behavioral Research* (New York: Holt, Rinehart, and Winston, 1967), p. 11.
15. I. Scheffler, *Science and Subjectivity* (New York: Bobbs-Merrill, 1967), pp. 37–38.
16. M. Brodbeck, "Models, Meaning, and Theories," in M. Brodbeck (ed.), *Readings in the Philosophy of the Social Sciences* (New York: Macmillan, 1968), p. 583.
17. A. Jacox, "Theory Construction in Nursing: an Overview," *Nurs Res* 23 (January–February 1974): p. 8, citing M. Blalock, *Theory Construction* (Englewood Cliffs, N.J.: Prentice-Hall, 1969), p. 11.
18. S.C. Roy, "Adaptation: Basis for Nursing Practice," *Nurs Outlook* 19 (April 1971): 254–57.
19. M. Brodbeck, "Models, Meaning, and Theories," in M. Brodbeck (ed.), *Readings in the Philosophy of the Social Sciences* (New York: Macmillan, 1968), p. 585.
20. *Ibid.,* p. 587.
21. *Ibid.,* pp. 583–85.
22. D. Orem, *Nursing: Concepts of Practice* (New York: McGraw-Hill, 1971), p. vii.
23. National League for Nursing, Department of Baccalaureate and Higher Degree Programs, *Revised Draft of Criteria for Appraisal of Baccalaureate and Higher Degree Programs in Nursing* (New York: 1976), p. 6.

24. *Ibid.*, p. 5.
25. M. Harms, *Development of a Conceptual Framework for a Nursing Curriculum*, papers presented at the 12th meeting of the Southern Regional Education Board Council on Collegiate Education for Nursing (Atlanta: Nursing Education Project, Southern Regional Board, 1969).
26. M. Gordon, "A Systematic Approach to Curriculum Revision," *Nurs Outlook* 22 (May 1974): 306–9.
27. C. Peterson, R. Hass, and M. Killalea, "Theoretical Framework for an Associate Degree Curriculum," *Nurs Outlook* 22 (May 1974): 321–24.
28. H. Brower and B. Baker, "Using the Adaptation Model in a Practitioner Curriculum," *Nurs Outlook* 24 (November 1976): 686–89.
29. P. Wagner, "Testing the Adaptation Model in Practice," *Nurs Outlook* 24 (November 1976): 682–85.
30. *Ibid.*, p. 683.
31. S.C. Roy, "Comment," *Nurs Outlook* 24 (November 1976): 691.
32. C. Hempel, *Philosophy of Natural Science* (Englewood Cliffs, N.J.: Prentice-Hall, 1966), p. 11.
33. *Ibid.*, pp. 11–12.
34. *Ibid.*, p. 12.
35. *Ibid.*, p. 13.
36. J. Dickoff, P. James, and E. Wiedenbach, "Theory in a Practice Discipline: Part II, Practice Oriented Research," *Nurs Res* 17 (May–June 1968): 545–54.
37. C. Lindeman and B. Van Aernam, "Nursing Intervention with the Presurgical Patient—the Effects of Structured and Unstructured Preoperative Teaching," *Nurs Res* 20 (July–August 1971): 319–32.
38. C. Lindeman, "Nursing Intervention with the Presurgical Patient," *Nurs Res* 21 (May–June 1972): 196–209.
39. J. Johnson, "Effects of Structuring Patients' Expectations on Their Reactions to Threatening Events," *Nurs Res* 21 (November–December 1971): 499–504.
40. J. Johnson and V. Rice, "Sensory and Distress Components of Pain," *Nurs Res* 23 (May–June 1974): 203–9.
41. J. Johnson, K. Kirchhoff, and M. Endress, "Altering Children's Distress Behavior During Orthopedic Cast Removal," *Nurs Res* 24 (November–December 1975): 404–10.
42. J. Johnson, "Effects of Structuring Patients' Expectations on Their Reactions to Threatening Events," *Nurs Res* 21 (November–December 1972): 499.
43. C. Lindeman and B. Van Aernam, "Nursing Intervention with the Presurgical Patient—the Effects of Structured and Unstructured Preoperative Teaching," *Nurs Res* 20 (July–August 1971): 321.
44. *Ibid.*, p. 500.
45. C. Hempel, *Philosophy of Natural Science* (Englewood Cliffs, N.J.: Prentice-Hall, 1966), p. 15.

CHAPTER SIX

ISSUES RELATED TO HUMAN SUBJECTS

Jean Hayter

Numerous issues exist today concerning the protection of human research subjects. Basic to many of these issues is the definition of research itself. Two widely disparate views prevail. One envisions research as the source of all good things, the ultimate means by which all problems will be solved. The other holds that research consists of experimentation which makes guinea pigs out of human beings, performs untold horrors without their knowledge or consent, and will ultimately yield products and techniques that man will be unable to control. Neither viewpoint is accurate, of course, but there is a modicum of truth in each. Progress generally does result from a research atti- tude, if not from systematic studies, and research clearly offers the best hope for increasing nursing knowledge. To expect that all problems will be solved by research is unrealistic, however, and might cause unjustified disappoint- ment in existing progress. Efforts to dispel the belief that research is a panacea for all problems—along with simultaneous efforts to foster realistic expectations of and respect for scientific investigations—will not only promote nursing research but will enhance the protection of human subjects.

The best way to eliminate the view of research as experimentation without due regard for human subjects is to demonstrate by high ethical standards and practices an acute sensitivity and concern for human welfare. Violation of human rights in the course of research, besides having negative effects on human subjects, is detrimental to trust in research in general, and arouses resistance which can impede future research. Since most progress does come from research, a ban on research would be unethical. But there is risk involved in any research. Nursing research, for instance, must of necessity involve human subjects, and it is not always easy to determine how human rights can best be protected or what the strict lines of control should be. It is this writer's intention to explore some of the issues pertaining to the protection of human rights, with the hope of stimulating thought and ultimately enhancing protection of the rights of human research subjects. Contrasting viewpoints will be presented and, whenever possible, guidelines will be given.

The writer will first attempt to give a perspective on the historical position of human rights in medical research. This will be followed by a systematic discussion of the essential rights of all human research subjects, as guaranteed by law, professional ethics, and common morality. The discussion will then move on to special problems concerning the necessity of informed consent, especially as this pertains to subjects who are mentally retarded, legally underage, or captive either physically or through social and economic circumstance. The author will then attempt to present the positions of those agencies and individuals that, through choice or by law, share the investigator's responsibility toward the protection of human subjects' rights. The chapter will then close with a discussion of the rights of the nurses themselves; as investigators, as participants through performance of their normal duties, and as subjects of research.

HISTORICAL PERSPECTIVES

Little attention has been given to protection of human subjects in the past. Without question, subjects have been sorely misused. The oldest world literature includes stories of prisoners being made freely available for human experimentation.[1] Jenner, who is honored as a giant in the history of medicine, deliberately exposed an eight-year-old child to cowpox so that he might try a new vaccine.[2] This kind of abuse wouldn't pass a modern review committee. This comment of an investigator shows the gross and open disregard for protection of human subjects as late as 1901: "Perhaps I should have first experimented upon animals, but calves—most suitable for these purposes— were difficult to obtain because of their cost and their keep."[3] Bernard,[4] a contemporary of Pasteur, made the first statement of ethical limits for studies involving humans. He said, "The principle . . . consists in never performing on man an experiment which might be harmful to him in any extent, even though the result might be highly advantageous to science." Encompassed in this simple statement is the ideal of today's ethical codes and also some of the most troublesome issues we face.

The need for more control over human experimentation became apparent especially after World War II, when the Nazi experiments were disclosed to the horror of the world. The Nuremberg judges formulated ten guidelines, a revision of which was adopted as the Declaration of Helsinki by the World Medical Assembly in 1964.[5] Those guidelines are in effect today but, as with any code, they are open to different interpretations and fail to provide for all circumstances. In 1966, USPHS issued guidelines for projects funded by that department, and that policy has now been extended to include all HEW-funded projects.[6] The American Nurses' Association's first guidelines for the protection of human research subjects were adopted in 1967.[7]

Marked changes have occurred in the past decade, both in the interpretation and implementation of ethical codes. These changes are probably due to the civil rights movement, an increasingly sophisticated and knowledgeable public, disclosure of political and legislative transgressions, and broad social reforms. Many investigators have used practices and procedures in the past, without misgivings, that they would not use today. In spite of these changes and the resultant strengthening of protective procedures, violations of human rights continue to occur. Two widely publicized examples have occurred recently—one involving the injection of live cancer cells into elderly and chronically ill patients without their knowledge,[8] and the other involving the deliberate exposure of mentally retarded children to infectious hepatitis.[9] Some people presume that well prepared professionals will act fairly and compassionately as a matter of course, and others believe experimentation without regard for the rights of individuals can significantly advance science. The Nazi experiments disprove both of these assumptions: highly qualified scholars then performed experiments with flagrant disregard for human rights, and the scientific benefits were minimal.[10]

History cannot be rewritten, but we can learn from it. In the overall effort to provide better nursing care to the public, investigators must keep in perspective the proper role of human subjects in scientific research. If a choice is to be made between research and human rights, human rights must always be given priority. People are more aware of their rights, and more self-protective, than they were even a decade ago, but in the final analysis the investigator is the one who must assume responsibility for the rights of human subjects. No doubt further ideological changes will occur in the future —nurses must be responsive to those changes as they occur and make certain their practices are compatible with society's ethical concepts.

RIGHTS OF HUMAN SUBJECTS

If human rights are to be adequately protected, attention must be given to the rights of informed consent, privacy, confidentiality-anonymity of data, protection from harm, and the right to refuse or withdraw from participation without recriminations. Each of these rights is discussed below.

Informed Consent

Informed consent has two components: recognition of self-determination, and thorough comprehension of the proposed participation. The freedom to choose what one will be and do is a vital part of being human. The right to self-determination is firmly established in America's constitution and moral beliefs. Every code of ethics applicable to research states that free consent is prerequisite to any human involvement. Philosophically, few if any professionals would deny that right. Nonetheless, in spite of codes and dictums, research without subjects' consent or knowledge was commonplace until recently, and there is considerable evidence that it still exists. Several factors help to explain why this is so.

The investigator may believe the patient will not be able to understand a scientific study. Health professionals have traditionally withheld information from patients about their diagnoses and treatments. In fact, the effect of treatment was believed to be partially dependent upon this secrecy, this element of mystery. Most of today's patients insist on knowing more about their illnesses and therapies, although there are still health professionals who prefer dependent, trusting patients to questioning, informed ones.

The investigator may not want to risk the patient's refusal. However, the subject's willing cooperation may increase the likelihood of a study's success. Some may think the patient's assent is so predictable that there is no need to ask. *Each individual reacts differently,* and no one can presume to decide for another what is awesome or appealing.

The investigator may believe it would frighten a patient to know that research is being done, or that it would decrease the patient's confidence in his care to imply that there are gaps in health care knowledge. The investigator might believe that asking a patient to sign his willingness to assume risk would create suspicion and fear. There is no better way to create suspicion—or to reinforce the all too prevalent public image of researchers as secretive and insensitive—than to have a person discover that he is, or was, a research subject without his knowledge.

An investigator s reluctance to seek a subject's consent may reflect dread of an open discussion. Some investigators do not want to admit that there are things they do not know. They avoid opportunities for unanswerable questions to be raised. Some investigators simply don't want to take the time to dispel a subject's doubts and fears. If an investigator believes that her request is justifiable, she should have no qualms about a free and open discussion concerning that request. There are, of course, large gaps in health care knowledge, and to think that an honest admission of this fact will shatter patient confidence is simply naive.

In the writer's experience, the most troublesome problems of consent in nursing studies stem from a belief that consent is only necessary under certain circumstances. An investigator may believe consent is necessary only when there is potential physical harm to the subject, or only when care will be altered in some way. The right to self-determination gives us the ability to decide whether we will be research subjects in *any* capacity. Confusion may result from lack of understanding of either self-determination or the research process. The investigator may feel uncomfortable about seeking the patient's consent, may somehow rationalize that no consent is needed. Sometimes it is argued that consent is unnecessary because everything being done for the patient would be done anyway, and the question arises, "What are we asking him to consent *to?*" The answer is often unequivocal—the patient is being asked to be a research subject. Whether his active participation is required or not, his consent is necessary if data are to be obtained from him for research purposes.

There are few things so complex or so technical that patients cannot understand them. The investigator must be able to explain things in terms comprehensible to the subject, or the research cannot be done. Most disciplines have ethical guidelines which mandate the subject's consent for research participation. This is clearly stated as a requirement in HEW policies[11] and in the American Nurses' Association's *Human Rights Guidelines for Nurses in Clinical and Other Research*[12]—investigators must do whatever is necessary to gain the subject's understanding and consent.

Unless the subject is fully informed in such a way that he can comprehend what will be done and why, it is impossible for him to be a willing subject. There is almost total agreement about that. The issues pertain, therefore, to the exact content and detail of the information to be dispersed.

One viewpoint is that subjects should be informed only in very general terms. Advocates of that position believe that most subjects don't have a scientist's interest in research and would only be frustrated or confused by full explanations. Alfidi's study[13] of patient preparation for diagnostic procedures provides some support for that viewpoint: 27 percent of the 107 subjects said explanations made them less comfortable, and only 69 percent said that all patients should receive a full explanation. Providing detailed explanations is also time-consuming, and it can be argued that if consent procedures are made impractical they will not be followed. Advocates of full explanations agree with this point, and say impatience, carelessness, and thoughtlessness are probably involved in inadequate explanations more frequently than deliberate disregard of patients' rights. However, considerable detail is necessary if patients are to have an adequate basis on which to make a decision, and the time required to do this must be considered secondary. There are numerous examples where subjects signed consent forms without fully comprehending the nature of the research. One such example is the widely publicized study in which neither teen-aged mental retardates nor their parents realized the girls were being sterilized. Another example is a study of a labor-inducing drug in which all 51 subjects gave written consent, although almost all of the subjects failed to understand at least one major aspect of the study, and 20 of the 51 did not even realize they were research subjects.[14]

Some investigators believe a lengthy exposition of possible risks might frighten subjects who would otherwise willingly agree; others counter by saying fear of the unknown is more anxiety-provoking than anticipating unpleasant events. Clearly, there can be two extremes concerning how much detail should be provided, and neither extreme is desirable. A lengthy exposition, with numerous minute details, can interfere with comprehension instead of fostering it. A balance between a vague, general statement and an unreasonably detailed explanation is more desirable. Some subjects will want more information than others—while there is certain basic information all subjects should have, explanations can be somewhat individualized according to a subject's interest and desire for information.

Most people agree that all subjects should have a clear, explicit explanation about each of the following aspects of the research: purpose and value of the project; procedures to be used and reasons they are necessary; the exact nature of the participant's role, including time and energy requirements; risks and benefits anticipated; any anticipated or potential loss of dignity or autonomy; anticipated pain or discomfort, psychological stress or embarrassment; and the way in which data will be handled and reported.[15]

Subjects who are being asked to contribute to a research effort have a right to know its purpose so that they can decide whether it is a cause they want to support. Each person has a right to decide which benevolent enterprises he will support. Subjects need to know whether they will be required to answer questions, take a test, fill out a questionnaire, permit observation, or participate in a new form of therapy. Since many nursing research subjects are sick, the energy requirement may be critical in the decision. For busy career persons, mothers with families, or students, contributing the necessary time may be quite a sacrifice. Knowing what is expected will provide a basis on which to make a decision.

Any potential risks should be explained realistically and objectively, including any potential discomforts, loss of dignity, or loss of self control. So far as possible, individuals should be exposed only to risks they have voluntarily chosen. What is perceived as a risk by one person may not be by another; and some people are willing to accept a degree of risk for the benefit of society, while others are not. In any event—even in the interest of new knowledge—investigators have no right to pick martyrs. Neither do they have the right to make any human being the means to an end, even if there is no discernible risk. Sometimes the risks are not fully known, and if that is the case the subject should be so informed. One further point, fully informing subjects reduces risk, for the subjects can then be alert to symptoms and can take precautions or immediate action as indicated.

Finally, the subject has a right to know the way in which data will be used. If more than one use is intended for the data, this should be explained and the subject's permission obtained for all intended uses. It is unethical to collect data for one stated purpose and use them for another. Here, too, there is a pragmatic as well as an ethical consideration: if subjects later discover that data they supplied or allowed to be obtained were used for an unexpected purpose, they may be reluctant to share information with health professionals again. That could not only have far-reaching effects on future research, but on health care and education as well.

The Right to Refuse or Withdraw from Participation

If a person has the right to give his consent to be a research subject, he also has the right to refuse. That option should be clearly stated, along with the promise that there will be no recriminations of any kind for refusal. And if a subject does choose not to participate, for whatever reason, that promise must be meticulously kept.

A variety of circumstances may threaten the right of refusal and make the subject feel that no viable choice exists. The subject may be intimidated by the investigator's credentials or prestigious position. An institutionalized patient's sense of power is reduced, and he is less inclined to question or dissent. Special problems exist if no other health care facility exists in the area, if the investigator is also in a provider role, or if the investigator is the patient's usual entry into the health care system. The patient may fear refusal will in some way affect the investigator's attitude toward him, or affect the attitude of other health care providers. This is far more likely to happen if the subject is receiving care without paying for it directly. He may feel that interest in him will be decreased or that his care will not be as good. Patients have been known to believe they could no longer receive health care if they chose not to be research subjects. The promise of monetary rewards, free care, or hospitalization in a special research unit can all be powerful influences and could be considered coercion.

Special caution is needed to make sure subjects do not feel intimidated into consent against their will. An attitude of concern and compassion by the investigator encourages free choice. An attempt can be made to increase the subject's sense of power by pointing out choices and emphasizing his right to arrive at a decision freely. If the investigator is herself aware of subtle pressures that may cause undue influence, she can more easily prevent resultant problems.

If the subject decides not to participate, that decision should be accepted uncritically, and the promise that there will be no recriminations must be adhered to strictly. No negative comments should be made to others, and no notations should be made on records which might influence other people negatively. Some have asked whether an investigator can honestly promise a subject the right to refuse without recrimination or bias when that investigator never has complete control over personnel and events. It is always possible that a member of the agency staff or someone unrelated to the study might be influenced by the subject's refusal. Perhaps a more common occurrence is that a patient will suspect his refusal made a difference and erroneously attribute future problems to it. In some instances it is possible to accord anonymity to those who refuse, and that might help. The best course of action is to try to establish a trust relationship with the patient, so that he will not be suspicious or fearful, and to scrupulously avoid any hint of displeasure if his choice is to not participate.

It is possible for the investigator to emphasize the subject's freedom of refusal so much that she inadvertently implies that a negative response is expected. If, on the other hand, the investigator states that the subject does have a choice but implies or allows the subject to infer some undesirable consequence of refusal, he may believe the right to refuse is inoperable. It is not easy for an investigator whose study depends on subjects to avoid hints or insinuations that the subject should consent. This is particularly true if the number of suitable subjects is limited, if time constraints cause pressure to secure a sample quickly, or if the refusal of some subjects introduces the problem of bias.

A subject may, at some time after consent, decide he wishes to discontinue his participation and withdraw from the study. His condition may change, he may find his involvement more tiring or more embarrassing than he anticipated, or circumstances may change to make his continuing participation inconvenient for him. Another possibility is that he may change his mind upon further reflection or upon talking with a friend or relative. In any of these circumstances, further discussion of the points of concern may take care of the matter, or it may be possible to relieve the inconvenience or discomfort the subject is experiencing. No actual pressure should be exerted to get him to continue in the study, however. If it seems that the subject finds his continued participation distasteful but is too embarrassed or too lacking in courage to say so, the investigator should discuss these hunches with the subject. If they prove valid, she should then support the subject in withdrawing from the study.

If the subject decides he wants the data he supplied or allowed to be collected about him removed from the study, it must be done, even if the subject's actual participation has ended. To insure that he knows ahead of time that his agreement to participate is not an irrevocable decision, he should be carefully apprised of his right to withdraw at any time. This can, of course, be very inconvenient and upsetting to an investigator who has invested considerable time and effort in data collection. The possibility of its happening can be greatly decreased by careful and honest explanations at the outset, but if it still happens, the choice is clear—the subject must be granted the right to withdraw without prejudice.

Privacy

The right to privacy includes privacy of one's thoughts, opinions, and physical presence, and privacy of one's records. An individual has the right to control the extent to which he shares himself with others. That includes the freedom to decide the time, extent, and general circumstances under which he will share his beliefs, attitudes, behavior, and presence with another. People have a right to be left alone if they wish and to withhold their thoughts from others.

Privacy, then, is a basic right that exists irrespective of whether research is in progress, and research provides no justification for violating that right. Since the extent to which individuals choose to share themselves with others varies with each person, and with the same person under different circumstances, it is essential that each subject be consulted about his willingness to share his privacy. One way of protecting human rights is to arrange a time and place that is convenient for the subject, if he has agreed to share his company with an investigator.

One aspect of privacy concerns the collection of data about an individual with no active involvement on his part. Data for many nursing studies could be collected by observation without the patient's knowledge or consent. This has been done in numerous instances, usually by a participant observer who was not identified as such. Even though nothing is required of the subject except allowing himself to be observed, it is a clear violation of the right of privacy to use him in a study without his informed consent. It may be that the events being observed are more or less public, but even so the individual must give his permission for the data to be used for research.

A few years ago it was commonplace to use such data collection tools as one-way mirrors, taped conversations, and concealed cameras or microphones without the subject's knowledge or consent. None of these measures meets today's ethical standards.[16] There are circumstances under which it is acceptable to postpone some aspects of the explanation, and these circumstances will be discussed later, but subjects should not be deceived by stating or allowing them to believe something that is not true. Such occurrences are partly responsible for the distrust and suspicion with which research and researchers are viewed. Subjects frequently do learn the truth, eventually, and the deception may prevent any kind of a trust relationship with them in the future. It could also cause them to be fearful or distrustful of health professionals generally, and the implications of that are tremendous.

The Privacy Act of 1974 brought under scrutiny the collection of psychological data through testing, in-depth interviews, or the use of drugs. These techniques may induce subjects to reveal more information about themselves than they wish to or are aware of revealing. Some tests or interview questions seem innocuous at first glance, but when interpreted are quite revealing. While the writer is not aware of any studies in which handwriting analyses or lie detector tests are used, these are other possibly misleading techniques. There is some question about the reliability and validity of some of these techniques, and others, which require interpretation for validity, can cause considerable psychological harm in the hands of an amateur. A basic concern, however, is the fact that an individual has the right to know what data are being obtained on him, the purpose of this data, and its use. The individual also has a right to refuse to supply or release the data.

Another aspect of privacy concerns the use of records for research. The Privacy Act specifies the right of access to one's own records and the right to prevent access of others to one's records.[17] Because nurses have free access to records as health care providers, teachers, or administrators, it is frequently hard for them to understand why the subject's permission is necessary before they can obtain or use data from records for research. If nursing roles are looked at separately, it is easier to understand. The nurse as health care provider uses data to plan the patient's care and make decisions for his welfare, and she has access to records for that purpose. If a nurse serves in a dual role, she still must obtain the patient's permission to use data from his health records for research purposes. She cannot use one role to gain access to data for another purpose. If the nurse investigator does not also have the function of providing care, she does not have legal access to the patient's records unless he grants that permission. Agency personnel are responsible for protecting health records, and the nurse investigator can expect that they will want assurance of the patient's permission before releasing records to her.

Since a subject gives his consent for data to be obtained and used only for a specific purpose, data collected for one study cannot be used for another unless the subject's consent is again secured. Investigators used to get all the information they could, in case they might find use for it in later studies. Therein lies another illustration of societal change and concomitant change in ethical standards. Such action would no longer be accepted by professional groups.

One reason for the Privacy Act was the development of technology which made possible the collection and rapid dissemination of masses of data without the knowledge or control of the subjects. Passage of a law does not guarantee elimination of the problem, however. Most people believe computers still pose a threat to privacy, but the extent of that threat is controversial. Some believe that computer-stored data constitutes an erosion of privacy which is impossible to control. Others say it is more difficult for the average person to obtain data from computers than to obtain information stored in traditional ways, since technical information is needed to get and interpret data from computers. Passwords and counterpasswords have been instituted to guard against unauthorized access to computer data, but that may only be further evidence of a problem. Decisions to share information are made by people, not computers. Sometimes only a select few are given the privilege of making those decisions. That might prevent unauthorized access to data, but it also might remove the individual's right to control access to and dissemination of information about himself.

Computers make it possible to assemble and disseminate large amounts of personal data in one central place. Trial printouts and extra copies of printouts might easily be pulled out of a wastebasket or allowed to fall into unauthorized hands. Recent talks of developing a national health file on everyone has enormous implications, some of which are frightening. There is a great need to plan precautions sufficient to prevent misuse or indiscriminate release of stored data.

Confidentiality—Anonymity of Data

Research subjects have a right to expect that data obtained about them will be handled confidentially—i.e., data will be available only to members of the research staff, and it will be reported anonymously. Complete confidentiality cannot be promised, for then the data could not be reported.

Confidential handling is an issue which causes some confusion. Sometimes health service personnel believe they should have access to all data about their patients, even data collected for research purposes. One needs only to remember that the subject gives consent for data to be obtained for a specific research purpose only, to realize that these data cannot be used except as necessary to accomplish that purpose. The investigator may be questioned by agency personnel about patients' responses. In fact, there have been instances in which staff personnel insisted that information be shared with them. It is advisable to inform agency personnel at the time arrangements are being made for data collection that the data will not be shared with them. A plan for sharing the research findings with agency personnel, developed and agreed upon before data collection begins, can essentially eliminate this problem.

Great care should be taken not to leave raw data where it might be seen by unauthorized persons. It should preferably be kept under lock and key while the study is in progress and then destroyed.

Sometimes, depending on the study design, complete anonymity can be promised. This means that nobody, not even the investigator, knows the respondent's identity. Anonymity should not be promised unless the research purpose can be accomplished without knowing the respondents' identities. If the research staff is large, identities can be coded and available only to one or two persons.

In studies involving mailed questionnaires, complete anonymity is possible but would make follow-up of non-respondents difficult. A reminder could be mailed to all subjects, asking those who had not responded to do so, but that adds considerable expense and reduces the effectiveness of the reminders. If complete anonymity *is* promised or implied, it is unethical to devise a code by which respondents' identities can be determined. Perhaps all readers have observed or heard of coding systems such as placing code numbers under the stamps on self-addressed envelopes or wording questions slightly differently on the separate questionnaires. As with other means of deception, trust is at stake, and loss of trust is more serious than any gains likely to accrue from it.

All would agree that anonymity should be assured in public reports. Contrary to the opinion of some, however, that involves considerably more than omitting the subjects' names. It requires reporting in such a way that no individual can be associated with any of the data by anyone who reads the report. One technique that helps to achieve anonymity in reporting is codifying data. Particularly when small numbers of individuals are involved, the categories should be carefully scrutinized to see if there is any way identity might be determined. If there are only a few respondents from a specific geographic location or age group or income group, for example, it might be possible to identify individuals on that basis. Sometimes anonymity can be achieved by combining categories. If no way can be found to maintain anonymity, the identifying data are simply not reported.

If subjects' cultural or socioeconomic backgrounds are different from that of the investigator, it is well to ask the subjects what data can be reported and how. Recognition of language, social customs, or folk lore might make it possible for identities to be determined, whereas that would not be apparent to an outsider.

Sometimes it is appropriate to protect the identity of an agency. That should be done unless knowledge of the setting is necessary to interpret results. There are times when disclosure of the agency would enable those familiar with it to identify individuals referred to anonymously in the report.

After the report is written, all data by which individuals could be identified should be destroyed. Someone else might find and misuse the data if they are retained, and the investigator is responsible for seeing that that does not happen. Research data do not have privileged legal status, and it is possible for them to be subpoenaed.[16] While this is unlikely, the possibility provides still another reason for destroying raw data as soon as possible. Even the manner of destroying data is important. They should not be dropped in a wastebasket, even if torn by hand previously, because of the danger of access by others before they reach a disposal system. Burning or shredding in a shredding machine is desirable.

Protection from Harm

Human subjects should be used only when risk of harm is minimal and when the research purpose can be accomplished in no other way. Since no research is risk free, the investigator is expected to adhere to sound scientific practices and to use all possible means to prevent or minimize harm. Explanations of possible risks, and the subject's willingness to accept them, in no way relieves the investigator of those responsibilities. There is little dissent about that. Issues associated with the subject's right to protection from harm center around a definition of harm, the degree of risk that is acceptable, and who should be exposed to what risk.

Most nursing research is descriptive, and the likelihood of physical harm is minimal where data are obtained about ongoing events without manipulation of an independent variable. As more nurses become prepared in research, and as the independent role of the nurse expands, one can predict that increasingly larger numbers of nursing studies will raise the issue of physical or physiologic risk.

Harm can take many shapes and forms, however. It can be an untoward reaction to a drug or failure of a wound to heal, but it can also be a fear of nurses that results from being asked unsettling questions by a nurse, doubts about one's adequacy as a parent which arise simply from being questioned about child rearing practices, or guilt feelings caused by questions about the living arrangements of elderly parents. Harm can mean fears or concerns about things the subject never knew existed until he was questioned about them; disturbing insights about oneself that come about through psychological testing or probing interviews; separation from one's family; or social isolation from lengthy hospitalization. Participating in a study may be safe as far as risk from physical harm, but it may be frightening to the patient. To ignore or deny the existence of such psychological and sociologic risks is to deprive the patient of precautions against these risks or help in dealing with them if they occur.

If subjects are to be protected from harm of any kind, the investigator must identify potential sources of harm and plan ways of avoiding them. Distress and psychological harm are made less likely by clear explanations, careful choice of words, an accepting attitude toward responses given, and prefacing questions about such things as child care practices with the statement that there are no right or wrong responses. If the study requires some loss of a subject's autonomy or control, the situation can be accorded dignity and handled compassionately.

A point of concern to some people is the use of an experimental design, because they believe it deprives some patients of effective treatment. If information existed to substantiate a treatment method's effectiveness, there would be no reason to study it. Therefore, one cannot say a patient is getting better (or worse) care by virtue of having an experimental treatment. Frequently risk can be decreased by improving the design. For example, a treatment method of known effectiveness could be used as a control instead of no treatment; if there is no method known to be effective, a traditional treatment method could be used as a control. Another possibility is to study the effect of positive instead of negative interventions, such as studying the effect of more teaching instead of less teaching. If any manipulation of variables would introduce risk, data could be collected about normal, ongoing events and an attempt made to determine correlations or cause-effect patterns from the data.

Sometimes there is financial risk involved in research participation, and that possibility should always be considered. The research might require prolongation of hospitalization and extra treatments, examinations, or supplies. Some financial losses are less obvious, but nevertheless directly attributable to the study; for example, transportation costs to a clinic, absences from work, or payment for a baby sitter. It is unjustifiable to expect or allow a research subject to incur additional expenses for his participation in a study. Potential sources of expense should be explored so that the investigator is aware of them.

The investigator tries to identify possible hazards and prevent them, but some risks are unpredictable and some will occur inevitably, even with preventive measures. If the investigator observes evidence of emotional distress she should take time to clarify the problem and/or help the subject work through his feelings. If any kind of undesirable effects occur which cannot be resolved immediately, the subject should be removed from the study. The usual practice is to provide whatever additional care the subject needs because of those effects. Some people are now raising questions about the legal liability of the investigator in such cases. The writer found no cases where a nurse was held liable for activities relating to research, but it does not seem compatible with human rights to leave subjects vulnerable. Malpractice insurance generally does not cover liabilities resulting from research activities, and it has been suggested that investigators obtain separate insurance coverage for that purpose.[18] With increasing litigation a current trend everywhere, there is no reason to believe research subjects are exempt. More important, this is an area where the rights of subjects seem to be inadequately protected.

The next issue, concerning the degree of risk that is acceptable, is particularly troublesome. Unfortunately, there have been instances where subjects were asked to assume considerable risk. In a recent study, 350 investigators described 424 studies carried out in two medical centers. It was concluded that in 18% of those studies the risk was not adequately counterbalanced by benefits, and in 8% the poor immediate risk-benefit ratio was not even compensated for by possible future benefits.[19] One could be an idealist and say that nothing is justified unless there is potential benefit with no chance of harm for the subject, but that would make all research with human subjects impossible. A more pragmatic approach is to say that likelihood of harm should be negligible unless the subject is likely to benefit significantly, and even then the subject should not be exposed to a significant amount of risk.

National Institutes of Health (NIH) guidelines for research involving human subjects describe the process of analyzing the risk–benefit ratio.[11] That consists essentially of assessing and comparing all potential risks and benefits, in order to decide whether the anticipated benefits justify anticipated risks. All potential risks, whether psychological, physical, social, or economic, must be identified and the likelihood and seriousness of those risks considered. One should then consider possible ways to avoid or minimize those risks. Potential benefits anticipated for either the subjects, other similar subjects, or society in general should be identified, and the risks and benefits compared. The term risk-benefit ratio sometimes gives the impression of a numerical ratio, but that is usually not possible. A verbal comparison of risks and benefits should accompany all grant applications, and all potential subjects should be given an explanation of anticipated risks and benefits. The current opinion is that no one should be asked to be a research subject unless the potential benefits either to the subjects or to society outweigh potential risks.

Another issue concerns deciding which subjects should be asked to assume risks. One viewpoint states that all subjects should have the specific problem being studied. This would eliminate healthy subjects completely, and would make it virtually impossible to establish norms. Deviations cannot be identified or interpreted unless there are norms with which to compare them. Some, however, say that sick people should not be asked to bear an additional burden and risk at a time when they are already vulnerable. The total exemption of ailing subjects from research is directly opposed to the position that all subjects should have the problem being studied. Here again the risk-benefit ratio is a useful guide. If the risk is negligible, and if the potential benefit to society is considerable, healthy subjects might be asked to participate. And, since those who have the problem being studied stand to gain the most if solutions are found, it seems justifiable to ask them to assume a somewhat higher risk.

The Golden Rule is often suggested as a guide for deciding whether a risk is justifiable for subjects: "Do unto others as you would have them do unto you." But expressing willingness to take the role of subject is not the same as being a subject. The investigator's own involvement in and motivation for the research can cause her to underestimate the risk and overestimate the benefit potential. At least 185 investigators have served as subjects for their own experiments and some have lost their lives as a result.[20] This raises the question of whether investigators should be permitted to assume a risk they may be unable to assess objectively. In 1968, the NIH issued a Code for Self-Experimentation "to provide the same safeguards for the investigator-subject as for the normal volunteer."[20] That code applies only to work done at NIH, Bethesda, Md. and not to all NIH-funded projects. No doubt some investigators feel that the imposition of such a policy would be an infringement upon their rights.

Securing Informed Consent

Obtaining a subject's informed consent is a critical aspect of protecting human rights and should be carried out meticulously and conscientiously. This involves the process in which the investigator explains the major aspects of the research as well as the prospective subject's involvement in it, and asks for the prospective subject's consent.

The first step is the construction of a consent form. This requires careful attention to insure that all essential elements are included and that it is worded unambiguously. Included in this form are: a statement of the purpose of the study; procedures to be followed; discomforts, risks, and benefits expected; alternative procedures (if any); an offer to answer any questions; a statement that the subject is free to withdraw without penalty; a statement assuring confidentiality-anonymity; and a statement that the subject is willing to participate in the study.[15] The intention to obtain data from records or to take photographs should be mentioned specifically. There are instances in which a statement should be included about uses which may *not* be made of data. For example, a study of the job satisfaction of nursing personnel might require a statement that the data supplied will not be used for evaluation purposes and will not be available to administrators. Space should be provided for the subject's signature, the signature of a witness, and the date. Beneath the subject's signature there should be a statement which the investigator signs, to the effect that she has explained to the subject the study in which he has agreed to participate.

The investigator should secure the subject's informed consent herself if at all possible. Sometimes, for convenience, consent forms are left with agency personnel. This is particularly tempting when consent of a relative or guardian must be obtained, and being present at the time they are present may require several trips or returning at inconvenient hours. The writer knows of an instance in which well-meaning agency personnel decided to tell the relative only that a picture would be taken, because they were afraid it would frighten the relative to know a study was being done. The investigator is responsible for insuring that informed consent is obtained, and it is preferable for her to secure it herself. Her signature as witness to the subject's signature is evidence that she was present when the consent form was signed.

The project should be explained in lay terms so that the subject is able to comprehend, and ask questions about, any aspect of the study. The greater the risk, the greater should be the patient's understanding. Words such as "experiment" and "manipulate" should be avoided, since they have different connotations to subjects than to investigators. Such terms as simple and routine should also be avoided, since procedures and techniques may seem simple and routine to the investigator but not to the subject. The subject should be told how he was selected for participation.

If appropriate, the investigator should specify services or opportunities which may be expected but will not be provided as part of the study. For instance, to avoid bias it is frequently inappropriate for the nurse investigator to provide care or advice to study subjects. An explanation of this at the outset will prevent false expectations. Clear understanding about the limits, as well as the benefits, of the subject's participation will do much to prevent later misunderstandings.

Sometimes a subject who from all indications would be able to make his own decision wishes to consult his attorney, a family member, or a trusted friend before deciding. Based upon the philosophy that the patient has a right to all information he regards as relevant, he should be encouraged to obtain such counsel. It might be advisable to offer to answer the questions of the person with whom he consults, since the subject may be unable to answer these questions himself.

An attempt should be made to verify that the subject does, in fact, comprehend the major aspects for which his consent is needed. This is usually done by asking the subject to express in his own words his understanding of what will be done and why. It has been proposed that a questionnaire be added to the consent form to verify and provide tangible evidence of the subject's comprehension.[15] Anticipation of the questionnaire might encourage the subject to listen more carefully and motivate the investigator to strive for a more fully informed subject.

Some people recommend giving a copy of the consent form to the subject to enable him to review his agreement with the investigator periodically and to compare his actual experiences with those he anticipated on the basis of explanations he was given.[15] It is generally recommended that a copy of the consent form be placed with the subject's records so that agency personnel will know the patient is a research subject. This is especially important if a special protocol is being carried out which requires the staff's cooperation. This practice also facilitates agency contact with the investigator in the event of a question about the project in the investigator's absence. On the other hand, putting a statement in the patient's file saying that he is a research subject could be construed as subtle pressure to participate, just as enclosing a statement that a subject refused could have a negative connotation. The investigator should definitely keep a copy of the consent form for her own files.

No doubt consent has been obtained on some occasions without the subject's understanding. One study showed that there was no more understanding among those who received a full explanation and gave written consent than among those who were approached and refused consent before receiving a specific explanation of the study.[21] Patients will sometimes consent, even at some inconvenience or discomfort to themselves, if they are approached agreeably. It is human nature to want to be helpful to others. Consent in some instances is no doubt based on blind trust and respect for the investigator, and no information is desired. Whether the subject wants information or not, whether it is difficult to secure his understanding or not, the investigator is obligated to satisfy herself that there is full and complete understanding and willingness to participate before the subject signs a consent form.

SPECIAL CIRCUMSTANCES THAT AFFECT HUMAN RIGHTS

Certain circumstances surrounding the research design or the research subjects require special attention to human rights. Included are subjects who are mentally or legally unable to give their own consent; subjects whose unique situation causes them to be more vulnerable to pressure or coercion; studies involving the use of animals; studies in which full disclosure at the outset would interfere with the research purpose; and studies which in some way alter the medical regimen. In this section each of these special circumstances will be discussed.

Mentally or Legally Incompetent Subjects

The Nuremberg Code states unequivocally that "voluntary consent of the human subject is absolutely essential."[22] Strict adherence to that would prohibit research involving the mentally ill, the mentally retarded, people who are unconscious, and children, and the consequences would be far-reaching. There has been considerable vacillation with regard to this issue and various stands have been taken. At this time there is no unanimity of opinion. General agreement seems to exist on two points: (1) persons who are unable to give their own informed consent should not be research subjects if other subjects can be used; and (2) the less able a person is to protect himself, the more vigilant the investigator must be in protecting him. There is also general agreement that inability to do studies of normal growth and development and studies about problems unique to these special groups would seriously interfere with progress in the health field.

It seems clear that a young child is mentally and emotionally incapable of weighing risks and benefits, resisting possible coercion, and reaching a reasoned decision about research participation. Until fairly recently, it was accepted practice for parents to give consent for their minor children to participate in research. Now, however, questions are being raised about the acceptability of parental consent. It has been said that parents do not own the child, they are merely his guardians until he can take care of himself.[23] It has also been said that a minor cannot abrogate his rights, that he merely preserves them, and upon reaching the age of legal majority he can sue for any wrongdoing that he perceives was done to him at an earlier age.[23] Some go so far as to propose that a mature person can sue for injuries sustained at any stage of his fetal existence, and investigators are advised to get parental consent in the presence of a third person if they do studies involving fetuses because of the seriousness of this threat.[24] No doubt recent legal and theological controversies about the issue of abortion have brought research involving fetuses under closer scrutiny. Resolution of these controversies is likely to bring further changes in the ethical standards for research involving fetuses, but it is impossible at this time to project the nature of those changes.

Most writers on the subject favor allowing parents to give consent for their children if there is no discernible risk and the child stands to benefit. Fletcher and O'Donnel say that if the child could consent, he would want what is beneficial to him.[5] Some say parents can give consent where there is negligible risk and potential benefit for others because one should support the things that are basically good.[5] Others counter by saying there is no way of knowing whether a child would wish to make a charitable contribution if he had adult understanding.[5] If one presumes that the decision rests on what the child wants, there is no way of knowing that he would want what is beneficial to him, would not want what is beneficial to others, or that he would or would not wish to take minimal risk where there is a potential for gain. A landmark decision was handed down by a Massachusetts judge, who ruled that a fourteen-year-old could be a kidney donor because he would suffer psychological harm if he were not permitted to do so.[25] This may bring about a revision of current thinking on the risk-benefit ratio.

Although profoundly different opinions do exist, and new interpretations or policies might be made at any time, prevailing opinion at this time seems to be that parental consent is acceptable for children if risk is negligible and if benefits can be expected to accrue to the child or to others with similar characteristics or situations. Even though parental consent is obtained, the child should be given as much of an explanation as he can comprehend and his approval should be sought and secured. Even with parental consent, the child should not be encouraged to participate against his will. Studies have shown that explanations to children in preparation for hospitalization help prevent emotional disturbances and loss of trust.[26] It seems reasonable to assume that explanations of research studies will have the same value.

Another issue pertaining to children concerns the age at which a child can grant consent. The age of 21 was originally chosen as the age of majority because that was the age at which a male had the skill and strength to engage in armed combat.[27] In some states 21 is still the age of legal majority, while in others it is 18. There has been little legal recognition that mature judgment develops gradually. There are numerous legal inconsistencies pertaining to age. A person is frequently considered capable of making his own legal decisions if he is in military service, married, or supporting himself, even though he is under the legal age of majority. Sometimes high school graduation or living away from home is taken as evidence of emancipation. There is no record of a court case where judgment was rendered against a physician for treating a minor over 15 on his own consent.[27] Schwartz found that even with careful explanations children under 11 are not aware of being research subjects.[26] The recent Supreme Court ruling that a minor does not need parental consent for an abortion is further evidence of the trend to allow minors to make decisions for themselves—at ages well below the legal age of majority. This issue is far from being resolved, and changes are occurring constantly. Current practice seems to be to obtain the parents' consent for minors except in those special circumstances outlined above, and to obtain the child's agreement according to his or her level of comprehension.

Certain circumstances seem to increase the risk of research participation for children. Schwartz found that there is more potential for psychological harm with children who are chronically ill, emotionally disturbed, or alienated from their families.[26] Beecher warns against discussing such delicate subjects as sexual attitudes with children, or asking them about occurrences in the home or about their parents' attitudes, for fear of placing the children in the position of spying on their parents.[28]

Consent for mentally ill, mentally retarded, or unconscious subjects, or for subjects who are mentally incompetent for any reason, raises issues similar to those discussed above. In all of these instances, there is a danger that comprehension will be only partial, and there may be no way to ascertain how much or how well the subject understands. In general, the same questions should be considered—whether there is discernible risk, whether the individual or others similar to him will benefit, and whether he is able to give his own consent in a completely informed way. In most instances, and to the degree to which that is possible, it is desirable to obtain informed consent from the subject and from a relative or guardian who is in a position to give legal consent for the subject.

Because of the stress experienced by dying patients, it can be argued that they are incapable of fully informed consent. Certain things specifically related to dying can only be studied with dying patients. Even so, no additional hardship should be imposed on dying patients without their approval. Some patients gain satisfaction from sharing their dying for the future benefit of others; it is one of the few remaining things they feel they can do. A point to keep in mind is that the subject's death might be somehow attributed to his research participation, even if there was no such actual relation.

If the study involves anesthetized subjects, or subjects who were unconscious and later regained consciousness, their consent can be obtained during a period when they are conscious. In one instance consent obtained from a patient who had been given a sedative was held to be invalid.[29] With this in mind, it seems advisable to ascertain that the patient has not had a central nervous system depressant before his consent is sought.

Aged persons need special consideration here for several reasons. First, the number of aged persons is rapidly increasing, and it is predicted that this number will increase still more in the coming years. That, plus growing interest in the field of gerontology, has resulted in a tremendous increase in research involving aged subjects. Finally, some but not all elderly persons are mentally incompetent due to degenerative diseases or acute illnesses and are unable to give true informed consent. If aged persons are unconscious, dying, or mentally incompetent for any reason, consent for them to be research subjects should be obtained in the same manner as for similar subjects of any other age. The chief difference with aged subjects is that they may be considered mentally incompetent simply because of their advanced age. Age alone does not cause mental incompetence. The aged subject should be assessed for the presence of factors which might make him unable to comprehend what he is being asked to do. Unless such factors exist, however, he can make his own decision as to whether he wishes to be a research subject. If the elderly person is a patient in a nursing home, economically deprived, or for some other reason in a dependent state, he may feel that he has no real choice. It is important for the investigator to first carefully explain to the subject that he does have the right to refuse, with no fear of prejudice because of his refusal, and then to do whatever is necessary to see that this right is protected.

The consent of mentally or legally incompetent subjects concerns an area where numerous legal and ethical changes have occurred in the recent past, and future directions are uncertain. Investigators should stay apprised of future changes as they occur.

Captive Subjects

There are circumstances under which a person might feel some compulsion to acquiesce when asked to be a research subject, whether that is his actual preference or not. He might believe rewards and benefits would accrue in return for his participation or that his refusal would create undesirable consequences. If either positive or negative pressures are in operation, it is difficult to insure the right of self-determination. Because of their unique life circumstances, prisoners, students, employees, or family members of the investigator, and residents of underdeveloped and low socioeconomic areas are particularly susceptible to these pressures. Special attention should be given to insure that these subjects are protected from genuine or perceived coercion. The main issue involved is whether members of these groups should ever be research subjects. Some people believe that existing subtle pressures and persuasions make it impossible for these people to give true informed consent. Others vehemently disagree and hold that willing subjects should not be denied the privilege of research participation.

Considerable attention has recently been focused on the misuse of prisoners. Studies have been cited in which prisoners were exposed to diseases and other considerable risks with little hopes of personal gain.[21] It seems clear that the risks to which some prisoners were exposed exceeded what is acceptable by today's ethical standards. Whether they were willing volunteers or were coerced is not clear. Some take the position that hopes of early parole, monetary rewards, special privileges, feelings of guilt, and an implicit expectation that prisoners will volunteer constitute undue influence. Others disagree and point out that participation breaks the monotony of prison life, boosts self-esteem at a time when prisoners have little opportunity to do that, and provides a link with the community at large and its values. Some believe the necessity to weigh the risks and benefits of the research encourages prisoners to give deliberate thought to their own purposes and values.

A study by Martin showed that prisoners' decisions about research participation were influenced more by monetary rewards and opportunity to gain the respect of others than by the risk incurred.[21] It is generally held that monetary rewards for research subjects should not be sufficiently large to influence their decisions. Most people believe that this should apply to prisoners, too, but a few say that since prisoners are unable to earn much money in prison they should not be denied that opportunity.[30]

Weighing all these factors, consensus seems to be that prisoners lose neither their right to participate in research nor their rights of self-determination, refusal to participate, and protection from harm by virtue of going to prison. In order to safeguard all those rights, prisoners should not be offered a reduced prison term, early parole, or special privileges, and monetary rewards, if any, should not be large enough to constitute coercion. In addition, a special effort should be made to avoid any implication that prisoners are expected to volunteer.

The possible abuse of prisoners has been given much attention, but other groups who are subject to similar subtle pressures are not as commonly recognized. For students, the prestige of a teacher, or of the research itself, the promise of extra points added to a grade, or even the promise of statements in their files saying that they participated in research can be forms of coercion. Even if no rewards are promised, and no negative actions threatened for nonparticipation, students may be reluctant to displease faculty members who are responsible for their continued education and on whom they will be dependent for references. The writer has been told of numerous instances in which students were asked to respond to questions, complete a form, or carry out an exercise which they believed to be part of a course requirement. Only later, sometimes when the study was reported, did they find out that they had been subjects in a study. This is a clear violation of subjects' rights, because they supplied information which was used for a study in which they did not agree to participate. Even if students are told verbally that informed consent is essential for research participation, they are likely to dismiss that as mere rhetoric if actual practice contradicts. Some faculty members take the position that being a research subject is a valuable learning experience, but others believe it is difficult to assure students that a genuine choice exists.

A similar predicament exists with regard to employees or family members of the investigator. There the possible pressures would be loyalty and respect for the investigator, the expectation that the investigator would not ask them to do anything risky, or the anticipation of favorable treatment for participation or negative reactions for nonparticipation. The writer has heard investigators report on pilot studies with employees or family members as subjects, which were carried out without any of the required review procedures or precautions. Several points are important to consider. Most office workers, laboratory assistants, and family members are insufficiently grounded in research to be aware of potential dangers, and it is the investigator's moral and legal responsibility to fully inform any potential subject of possible hazards. Even more distressing, the fact that an investigator would omit the customary precautions for these subjects suggests that she considers the precautions unnecessary. This brings to mind again the fundamental concept that no procedure or requirement can insure the protection of human rights unless the investigator has integrity.

Nurse researchers must be very concerned about subjects from underdeveloped or low socioeconomic areas. Most medical centers are in large urban areas, and that is where most nursing research is done. Medical centers draw heavily on patients with limited funds or limited access to health care. There is likely to be a large proportion of elderly and socioeconomically and culturally deprived individuals in such populations. Not only is the problem of an unrepresentative sample a troublesome one, but the dependent, power-deficient position of such patients makes them much more vulnerable to coercion. They may believe they have no choice but to comply with whatever request is made of them. They may be unaware that risk is involved, and explanations of risks may be overshadowed in their minds by their concern for continued health care. Unsophisticated people may be so impressed with descriptions of new and improved methods of care that casually mentioned risks or possible consequences seem unimportant to them. It seems clear that disadvantaged, socially and economically deprived persons have been overused as research subjects and that in some instances they have been misused.

Residents of underdeveloped areas, such as Appalachia, and residents of urban ghettos have been studied ad infinitum, sometimes with little regard for possible harmful consequences. Some investigators have collected data in underdeveloped areas and have then used this data for their own purposes, without insuring that those who supplied the data in some way benefitted. A common problem with studies involving underdeveloped areas and low socioeconomic groups is that a project is started with grant funds and then terminated when the grant funds expire. Considerable harm can result from short-term projects unless plans are made from the beginning for the project's systematic termination or for its continuation without grant funds.

As with prisoners, these groups should not be denied the privilege of participating in research, but neither should they be enticed to participate by the subtle pressures to which they are uniquely susceptible. Because of the increased likelihood of harmful effects as a result of research participation, as well as the great danger that the subjects might not fully comprehend the risks involved, a special effort must be made to inform them fully and to afford them ample protection. There is always some danger of subtle pressure with any potential research subject, but the danger is clearly greater with these groups. Even if these guidelines were adhered to meticulously, there would still be a nagging doubt about whether such factors as fear of negative consequences, fear of displeasing a person with perceived power, or anticipation of rewards from participation might create subtle pressure. Perhaps all an investigator can do is to be sensitive to the possibility of such pressures, and alert to their existence, and to use all reasonable precautions to avoid undue influence on subjects' decision. Perhaps then there will be no true captive subjects.

Animal Subjects

Perhaps the major issue pertaining to animal subjects is whether animal studies are appropriate for nurse investigators. Some say there is such an urgency for clinical nursing research, and so little nursing research being done, that all research efforts should be directed toward findings with immediate applicability to practice. Others say that research is possible with animal subjects which would never be possible with human subjects and that findings from those studies are applicable and far-reaching. Only a few studies have been done by nurse investigators using animal subjects. No doubt there will be more in the future as nursing's overall emphasis on research increases.

If studies are done with animal subjects, the investigator must insure that they are humanely treated. HEW regulations specify that animals used for research purposes must be properly and adequately cared for and that their suffering, discomfort, and distress must be kept to a minimum.[31] The animals should be kept in suitable facilities, properly fed, supplied with water, and exercised or permitted to exercise. HEW policy further states that experimental animals should be used in research only when there are no other feasible means to accomplish the purpose.[31]

If Full Disclosure Would Alter Outcomes

There are numerous instances in which full disclosure of some aspect of the research would alter the subject's response and/or make it impossible for the research purpose to be accomplished. A few examples will clarify this problem: (1) studies of honesty are possible only when the subjects do not know honesty is the characteristic being studied; (2) disclosure of purpose in a study to determine relationships between parent and child or between spouses would alter those relationships; and (3) if the purpose is to study reactions to an emergency, full disclosure would remove the surprise element which is a prime factor in emergencies.

It is acceptable to postpone explanation of some aspects of the research if subjects are informed that some information is being withheld and that debriefing will be done later. Deception, unlike the withholding of information, means that false information is given or implied. Sometimes false information is not actually given but the subject is led to believe, or allowed to believe, something which is not true. Deception occurs just as surely when an untruth is implied as when it is stated outright. Although some people consider it acceptable to deceive or mislead a subject as long as the deception is revealed later, most people consider deception in any form unconscionable. A much quoted example of deception is a study in which mothers were told that their children were to be observed and that the mothers' help was needed to get the children to follow certain instructions. The study was, in fact, on mother-child relationships, and the mothers, not the children, were the research subjects.[32] Another example concerns numerous studies of pain in which inert substances were administered while subjects were told they were receiving a drug to relieve pain. In the first example, loss of dignity and decreased self-esteem are likely to have resulted. In the second example there is loss of trust and unnecessary pain—the patients might also suffer from worry and mental anguish in an attempt to understand why the "drug" does not relieve their pain, and might think their conditions have gotten worse. Ethical standards dictate that no patient should be allowed to experience avoidable pain or suffering, whether that suffering is mental or physical.

It seems, therefore, that outright deception should not be used in research. Deception violates the respect and trust which are basic to all human interactions. It can create anxiety, frustration, embarrassment, and decreased self-esteem. The suspicion caused by deliberate falsification can result in a wariness that interferes with subsequent studies in which the subjects might be involved. Even more serious, this loss of trust could be carried over into other aspects of their lives. Studies which involve deception can result in rejection of essential health care and general mistrust of all health professionals.

Delaying certain explanations, with the subject's knowledge, is permissible and sometimes necessary. It may be done more frequently than necessary, however. One study showed that in 19.3% of 457 studies some part of the explanation was withheld.[32] Guidelines for doing studies in which full disclosure in advance is not possible center around two concepts: informing subjects that some aspects of the research process are being withheld and debriefing.

Only information which would invalidate a study's findings should be withheld, and subjects should be told that certain information cannot be revealed until later. In some studies, subjects could be made aware that certain data will be obtained without their prior knowledge. They can often be told the area of the study and the general nature of their involvement. Sometimes subjects can be told about their projected involvement without reasons for it. Under certain circumstances it is appropriate to tell subjects that they will not be asked to do anything that opposes their moral principles or that would embarrass them. When subjects are told that some information must be temporarily withheld, definite plans should be made for debriefing.

Debriefing consists of a complete disclosure of all information previously withheld, an explanation of why the information could not be given before, a sincere statement by the investigator that she regrets the necessity to withhold information, and an offer to answer any of the subject's questions. If the impression is conveyed that the investigator enjoyed the deception, no amount of explanation will erase the resentment and feeling of having been tricked. Debriefing consists of more than supplying the information that was withheld. It is an attempt to help the subject work through his feelings about the study so that he will feel good about himself and about the study in which he participated.[32] Debriefing frequently takes longer than the actual data collection.

Debriefing should be done before the findings are reported. There may be situations in which withheld information affects the subject's decision to participate. When full disclosure occurs, he may decide he wishes the data he supplied, or data collected about him, removed from the study. If this is the case, the investigator is ethically bound to destroy that data and may not use it.

There are times when no kind of explanation can be given to subjects in advance. An example is a study of reactions to an emergency. It is not known ahead of time who will be involved or who will be present when an emergency occurs. Under such circumstances it is acceptable to make observations without the subject's consent, but his informed consent must be obtained before the data are used. As soon after the data collection as possible, the study should be fully explained to subjects and the observations that were made of them should be reviewed. If they want to give their consent for use of the data, they should give their written informed consent at that time (after the previously described procedure). If the subjects do not consent, the data cannot be used and must be destroyed.

If Medical Regimen Would Be Affected

There are times when a nursing study would affect or require alteration of a medical plan of treatment. For example, in a study pertaining to pain relief the independent variable might be distraction, positioning, or some means to help the patient relax, all measures that fall within the realm of nursing, but unless some control is placed on the use of analgesics, it becomes difficult to assess the effect of the independent variable. Another example might be a comparison of two different nursing methods to promote healing of decubitus ulcers. Even though the treatment methods might consist of some combination of massage, cleansing, and relief of pressure—all within the purview of nursing responsibility—success of the study would be greatly enhanced by the physician's refraining from ordering topically applied medications. If a nursing study affects or would be altered by a medical regimen, the investigator should obtain the physician's approval for whatever adjustment of the medical regimen is needed.

If the design for a nursing study requires the administration of a certain drug, the drug must be prescribed by a physician or it cannot be administered. Nurses do not have the authority to prescribe drugs, and being the investigator of a clinical nursing study does not alter that fact. Therefore the physician's collaboration must be sought. The nurse investigator should tell the physician why the research requires that subjects have a certain drug or specific amounts of a drug, or that a drug be withheld. The decision about whether to prescribe the drug is ultimately the physician's, of course, just as are all other aspects of the medical regimen.

Unless a nursing study affects the medical regimen or would be affected by it, it is not necessary to request the physician's approval. Health professionals do not customarily seek each other's permission to have access to patients or patients' records, nor is this necessary, since no one professional group has the right to grant or deny access to other health professionals. If subjects are under the care of a physician, he or she should be informed that a nursing study is planned and given information about the purpose and nature of the study, just as a nurse would want to know about a medical study that involves patients under her care. Seeking approval connotes the alternatives of assenting or dissenting; informing does not give that connotation.

SHARED RESPONSIBILITY FOR HUMAN RIGHTS

There is general agreement that the best safeguard of subjects' rights is an investigator who has integrity, professional expertise, a sense of responsibility, and compassion for human subjects. Not all investigators possess these humanitarian characteristics, however, and even if they do, that alone is inadequate to insure adequate protection of subjects' rights. This section includes a discussion of some current practices by which peers, funding agencies, health service agencies, and journal editorial boards share responsibility with investigators for protection of human rights.

It was pointed out earlier that the investigator's own involvement in the research may interfere with his objectivity, but there is evidence that more is involved than lack of objectivity. Lally[33] found that the "compassionate physician is not found among physician-researchers as often as some have suggested." He reports finding a connection between compassion and the quality, frequency, and duration of interactions between researchers and subjects. Beecher[34] reported several well documented instances in which there was flagrant disregard of human rights, and he speculates that this occurs much more frequently than is known. Barber[19] suggests that the reason may be lack of attention to ethical standards in educational programs. He found that only 13% of over 300 physicians had had even a single lecture devoted to the ethical issues involved in research with human subjects. The writer found no information about the presence or absence of compassion among nurse-researchers or about their educational preparation concerning ethics. One would like to think the picture is different for nurses than for physicians, but there is no evidence to this effect.

Institutional Peer Review Committees

Because of increasing concern about human rights, the United States Public Health Service (USPHS) issued a policy in 1966 requiring approval by a peer review committee, at the institution requesting funds, for all proposals involving the use of human subjects.[35] This policy now applies to all HEW-supported research. Most health service and educational institutions also have a policy requiring that all research involving human subjects, done in or under the purview of that institution, must be approved by a peer review committee.

While there are usually representatives from the social, biological, and health sciences, peer review committee membership is not limited to professionals. An important point to mention is that committee membership requires no knowledge of research or health care. HEW regulations now mandate outside representation on such committees.[36] Justice Holmes said that our jury system keeps the law in touch with public opinion.[2] Lay membership can do that for peer review committees. Also frequently included are a chaplain and a hospital administrator. This committee composition is intended to provide a system in which an objective group, with different perspectives and biases, can exercise group judgment about the adequacy of the protection of human rights in specific studies.

Numerous issues exist concerning the purposes, effectiveness, and limitations of peer review committees, and there is general agreement that some changes are needed. Deciding which changes would improve the situation is not as easy. Many of the issues center around two differing viewpoints. One view is of the committee as a policing group, looking over investigators' shoulders to see whether they are behaving; the other is a view of the committee as a source of help, part of a system of checks and balances, a group with which investigators can share the risks involved in research.

The committee can without question serve an educational function and be a source of help for investigators. It can serve a sensitizing function by calling attention to human rights and potential problems pertaining to them. A group with fresh outlooks about a problem and diverse experiences to draw from may be able to generate ideas that the investigator would never have envisioned. Some investigators welcome this help and are grateful for suggestions. Others believe it interferes with their own individual creativity and judgment. Some believe the requirement of external controls implies that their own professional conduct is in question. They particularly resent the fact that a committee assesses and passes judgment about their abilities to accept the responsibility for human rights and to carry out the projects they propose. The fact that non-scientists and non-professionals are exercising that judgment adds fuel to the flames.

The way a given committee or institution interprets the committee's purpose makes considerable difference in viewing the issues. According to HEW regulations, peer review committees have the express purpose of protecting the rights and welfare of human subjects.[11] That implies that the committee's function is limited to those aspects that pertain to protection of human subjects, which is the most frequently stated interpretation.[37] With that purpose in mind, a committee would not concern itself with the scientific soundness of research design except as it pertains to human rights. Gray[14] reasons, on the other hand, that the risk-benefit ratio cannot be assessed, and judgment made as to whether there would be sufficient valid results to justify subject participation, unless the scientific soundness of the research design is evaluated. He also reports, however, that one peer review committee whose activities he studied intensively had considerable doubt about criticizing research designs and that they rarely concerned themselves with that function. If the committee's function does extend to the research design, then the membership of those with no preparation in health care or research is questionable. Investigators, too, have rights, and giving authority to make decisions about research design to those with no research competence raises questions about these rights. Gray's conclusion that risk-benefit ratio cannot be assessed without analysis of the complete research design seems to negate the position that a patient, who is usually completely unable to analyze or evaluate a research design, could assess risks and projected benefits and arrive at a reasoned judgment about whether he wishes to be a subject.

Still a third viewpoint is held about the purpose of peer review committees. Gray[14] quotes Katz as saying that the USPHS policy grew out of fear of congressional displeasure should anything go wrong in USPHS-funded research. Gray concludes that the real purpose of the policy that founded review committees is to protect researchers and funding agencies or, stated another way, that the policy is intended to convince potential critics that its stated goal is being met. It is hard to believe that that was the sole intended purpose of the policy, but that may be its major accomplishment. Clearly, there are problems due to noncompliance with and misuse of the policy, as well as lack of control over some aspects very important to human rights. The two most troublesome problems in relation to peer review committees center around inadequate surveillance of research activities and lack of monitoring of the committee's functioning.

Failure to monitor all research results in many studies being done without their being submitted to the institution's peer review committee. In Barber's study, 10% of the respondents stated that their institution's committee reviewed only projects with outside funding, and 8% stated that at least one of their own studies had not been reviewed.[19] Barker found that 15% of the 293 institutions studied fail to review all research involving humans. One person reported hospitalized patients being studied without their consent and later being billed for the experimental procedures.[38]

HEW regulations say that committees are to review the research at appropriate intervals and in such a way as to assure that human rights are being protected.[39] This statement is vague, and the charge is unclear. HEW policy does specify that records must be kept of safeguards taken and that HEW must be notified of any ethical problems that develop.[39] The only action that committees commonly take to monitor ongoing research is to ask the investigator to notify the committee of any ethical problems and to supply an annual written statement saying that the research is being carried out as planned. In most instances, therefore, the only assurances of protection of human rights are a written plan of what actions are intended and a written statement that those actions are being done.

There is not much recourse for those who choose not to follow approved plans either. HEW policy states that the grant will be terminated and future funds banned if the regulations are not followed.[36] But in a system which operates on the assumption of good faith, failure to comply would probably never be discovered. Gray reports on interviews with 15 investigators, two of whom freely admit that they decided not to get subjects' informed consent or to tell them they were involved in research, even though the peer review committee had stated that written informed consent must be obtained.[14] About the only restraint on investigators when no grant funds are involved is their desire for the respect of their peers. Barber[19] reports an interesting study, in which he asked 350 investigators whether or not they would approve certain hypothetical studies. Investigators who were unsuccessful and striving for recognition, or those who were not considered by their peers to have scientific excellence, were found to be the most likely to approve studies with unfavorable risk-benefit ratios.

Others have pointed to the system of rewards and recognition as an important determinant of concern for human rights. This raises the question of whether giving more positive recognition for protection of human rights might not be a good way of safeguarding those rights. At best, there is all too little attention paid to positive reinforcement for health professionals in competitive, high pressure work situations. It seems possible that the review process can itself serve as positive reinforcement for investigators, a means of acknowledging that they are doing a worthwhile task well and that they are exercising great care to insure that human rights are protected. Both human subjects and human investigators would benefit from that approach.

The second major problem area with peer review committees concerns the lack of monitoring and evaluation of the committee's functioning. Each committee operates in relative isolation, with little monitoring, coordination, or review of its operation. The status interests, and number of the committee members all affect committee functioning. If the committee is very large, it is cumbersome and progress is slow. The review process is time-consuming at best, but further delays can be discouraging and inconvenient to investigators. If the committee size is small, one powerful member, or a member with a great deal of status, can exert undue control. Sometimes committees are dominated by physicians. Numerous instances exist in which there is no nurse member at all. The American Nurses' Association (ANA) has taken the position that all occupations likely to be involved in research should be represented on the committee.[40] Committee members may feel bound by professional loyalties to support the proposals of people in their own specific disciplines. On the other hand, jealousy or departmental competitiveness may cause committee members to be unduly critical of proposals submitted by a colleague. Having representatives from a variety of disciplines, as well as lay members, helps to reduce a tendency to back scratching or vindictiveness. Sometimes lay members are appointed for political reasons rather than for concern about human rights. This is obviously inappropriate.

One additional point about committee structure—a peer review committee must have both independence and authority to act, and should report directly to the administrative officer in charge of the institution, so that there will be no pressure to make certain kinds of decisions. Only then will the committee have the true ability to raise questions about or reject a proposal submitted by a highly respected member of the staff or by a person in a position of power. But that very autonomy creates the problem of the committee's actions being shielded from scrutiny and criticism. The committee is composed of individuals who are presumably interested in human welfare, but they, too, are human beings with vested interests and biases and human failings. They may use their positions on the committee to accomplish purposes far removed from human rights, and because of the committee's insulated position even gross injustices could go undetected. The committee could be a subtle means of exerting control over a variety of circumstances in the institution, such as who does research, whose work is facilitated and whose delayed, what problems are emphasized in the institution's research efforts, how soft money is spent, and who submits projects for what purposes to outside agencies for funding. Batey[41] calls attention to this problem and says, "Human rights protection is a legitimate and appropriate concern, but I believe more and more that it is used as a guise for other purposes—a form of power over the scientific process and researchers."

Some changes which might lessen these problems follow. (1) Summaries of decisions made, with studies reported anonymously, could be written and shared with other professionals. This would provide precedents on which other committees could base decisions, and it is one way to reduce the variance in the decisions of different committees. (2) A system for appeal could be instituted so that any investigator who believed unnecessary delay occurred or that the decision of a committee was unfair or prejudicial could request a second independent review. (3) More careful thought could be given to the method of committee selection. Both administrative appointments and appointments involving volunteers could cause problems. Administrative appointments might be used as a means of controlling the committee, and those who wished to exert control might be more inclined to volunteer. It is highly desirable that people who serve on these committees be fair-minded, competent individuals who have enough self-confidence and ego strength to avoid undue influence by others. Election of members by those people they will represent seems preferable. Also, to prevent the build-up of power groups, it is desirable that committee members serve only for a limited period of time.

Funding Agency Staff and Review Committees

Basically the same problems and concerns exist with the review boards of funding agencies as with those of an institution. There is probably less likelihood of power cliques, colleague coercion, and personal vendettas on committees of funding agencies, since these committees are made up of people from widely scattered areas. Also, decisions of funding agencies, particularly governmental agencies, are more available for public scrutiny than those of institutional committees. On the other hand, the stakes are higher in funding agency committees, and there are probably more efforts to sway decisions. There is also more potential power to influence not only selection of research projects, but the whole direction of research efforts on a nationwide basis. Those committees should be, and generally are, filled by the most capable, most highly principled persons available.

The functioning of a governmental committee is of necessity complex. Procedures should be kept as simple as possible, and the time involved for decision making should be reduced as much as possible, so that bureaucratic regulations and delays do not become so burdensome as to discourage research. Much valuable assistance is available from funding agency staffs, and the value of that help should not be discounted. Once a project is approved by such a committee, the investigator has the security of knowing his proposal has been scrutinized by experts and found to be worthwhile. He knows that that agency will share with him the responsibility for attesting to the proposal's soundness and will help interpret its value as the need arises.

Health Service Agency Staff

Some health service agencies have a peer review committee and some do not. If the agency is part of a university, there is usually no separate committee to review projects involving patients. Batey[41] clarifies agency responsibilities by saying that they should have reasonable control over what happens in the agency, and that they are responsible for the patient's care and welfare but not for the ethics of the research study. Batey further states that there is a need for conditions under which the freedom of inquiry can exist, and she cautions that we need principles for the protection of investigators, too. Agency personnel do have responsibility for the setting in which clinical nursing research occurs, and they are charged with safeguarding the welfare of patients while they are there. Whether the agency has a review committee or not, there should be a clear understanding between agency staff and the investigator about the purpose of the research and in general when and how the data will be collected. Agency personnel are frequently questioned about research. If there has been open communication and clear understanding about the study in advance, they can share the responsibility for interpreting the research.

Journal Editorial Boards

Finally, the protection of human rights is shared by journal editorial boards. Few investigators would carry out studies if they thought their reports would not be published. Editors are expected to use their influence to promote high ethical standards. Many editorial boards, that of *Nursing Research* among them, have agreed not to publish research reports unless they adhere to ethical standards.[42] The most stringent editorial policies the writer is aware of are those adopted by the *Council of Biology* editors. They require submission of a photocopy of the peer review committee's approval statement and a statement saying that the committee approved the proposal. If there is any concern, the committee's guidelines and a copy of the proposal the committee approved are requested. If there is concern about how the study was carried out, the committee chairman is asked to state that he is satisfied that the research was carried out in an ethical manner.[43] Some have suggested that studies which lacked adequate protection of human rights should be published and that attention should be called to the ethical lapse.[43]

When the report is ready for publication it is too late to correct any wrongs that might have been done, but the knowledge that a work will not be published without evidence of human rights protection serves as an effective deterrent to carelessness or neglect. Taking proper precautions is also reinforced when the editorial board reviews and approves a report.

RIGHTS AND RESPONSIBILITIES OF NURSES IN VARIOUS ROLES

The Nurse as Investigator

The ANA's guidelines state that qualified nurses have a right to do research and to have access to resources necessary for scientific investigations.[44] Some people find it hard to view nurses in the role of investigator and disagree with that position. Medicine's dominance over nursing practice sometimes carries over to research efforts, so that physicians think they should be in charge of or give direction to nursing research. On the other hand, physicians may find it acceptable for nurses to do research but believe it is the physician's prerogative to say whether certain patients can or cannot be subjects. Sample selection dependent on a physician's approval, with the connotation that he will sometimes withhold approval, could result in a biased sample and could, in fact, make the study impossible. Nurses who are qualified in research have a clear and inviolable right to plan and direct nursing research, as do investigators from other disciplines.

The writer's recent experience has been that members of other disciplines may be more likely than physicians to hold a stereotyped view of the nurse as the physician's assistant. Perhaps competent, well prepared nurses are beginning to alter the opinions of those with whom they come in contact.

It is important for nurses to demonstrate their ability and willingness to assume the responsibilities that research entails. Nurses who engage in research must be sure that they are adequately prepared to carry out high quality research without threat of jeopardizing human rights. That seems so irrefutable as to make it sound trite, but it is not viewed as irrefutable by some nurses. Viewpoints on this issue are contradictory and a bit confusing. Some say that all nurses are researchers, while others say almost nothing pertaining to clinical nursing is research. The fact that both clinical nursing research and clinical nursing practice pertain to nursing does not make them synonymous. Perhaps the confusion is partly due to failure of some nurses to understand how research differs from problem solving. It could also be that in some instances nurses, like some investigators reported in literature, simply do not want to go through the process of committee review, consent of subjects, etc., required for research and have found a way to satisfy themselves that it is unnecessary. Whatever the reason for the confusion of differing viewpoints, one thing seems clear. Competence in nursing research does require preparation for research, just as surely as competence in nursing practice requires preparation. To promulgate the viewpoint that all nurses are researchers, or to encourage or do research without essential qualifications, is a threat to the subjects' human rights and a threat to the right of nurses who are properly prepared to do research.

The Nurse as Participator in Research

Nurses are frequently expected to collect data or give medications or treatments as part of investigations being carried out by someone else. The major issue involved is how much information the nurse needs in order to participate in this manner. There have been many cases in which nurses were not informed that a study was being done, and many others in which they were told only that a new drug was being tried or that certain data were to be collected. Nurses who are participators in research need to be fully informed about the potential risks of measures they carry out, ways of recognizing when risk is present, and proper actions to take to counteract undesirable effects. This is important whether the investigator is a nurse or a non-nurse. A nurse participator who is not fully informed about the investigation may inadvertently bias the results. If she does not know the expected drug responses and symptoms of untoward and expected effects, she cannot carry out her legal and ethical responsibilities to observe the patient. If an experimental drug is being used, she should know the average dose, therapeutic and toxic effects, and precautions to be used. This information must be available for every drug used with humans, so it is not a question of the information's not being available.

The ANA's guidelines suggest that potential research participation should be discussed at the time a nurse accepts a position. They also specify that if employment is not accepted with the expectation of research participation as a requirement, the nurse should have the option of not participating.[45]

Particularly when controversial treatment methods such as abortion or heart transplantation are being studied, the question is raised as to whether nurses are free to refuse to participate. Milgram's study, as cited by Savard,[46] is interesting to review in that connection. She asked subjects to carry out a procedure which they thought was painful to other people, in an attempt to determine whether they would inflict pain as instructed. She found that most of the subjects were very perturbed because they were inflicting pain but, nevertheless, they kept on doing as instructed. There is no way of knowing how frequently nurses are asked to participate in studies of which they disapprove. Neither is there knowledge about how frequently nurses continue doing as they are instructed in spite of guilt or psychological turmoil. No nurse can be expected to engage in a study which is against her own ethical or moral principles. Furthermore, if she disapproves of the study, she may bias the results, because her attitude is likely to be apparent to subjects.

Nurses as Research Subjects

If nurses are research subjects, they have a right to expect that their rights will be fully protected. All the precautions and procedures discussed earlier in ths chapter are applicable to the nurse subject just as they are to any other subject. Most investigators are sensitive to the need to protect patient rights, but they do not always recognize that every human research subject, in whatever capacity, has those same rights. Many nurses have been sensitized to this problem because of the numerous studies of nurses carried out by other disciplines, sometimes without the nurses' knowledge or consent. If a study involves observing the care given by nurses, comparing taped and oral reports, obtaining nurses' opinions about working conditions or salaries, or anything in which data are collected from or about nurses, informed consent of the nurses involved must be obtained. This seems to be uncontroversial, but it is frequently omitted thoughtlessly. Nurse investigators should therefore remind themselves that any research involving human subjects requires that the rights of those human subjects be fully protected. Nurses who are asked to participate or who find themselves being involved in studies should insist that all necessary measures be taken to protect their rights.

SUMMARY

In this chapter the writer has attempted to analyze various issues pertaining to human subjects and to show why the protection of human rights must be accorded the highest priority in nursing research. As stated at the outset, it is not always easy to determine how human rights can best be protected.

There are certain requirements, established by law or organizational policies, that must be met. Professional codes and ethical standards give guidance for making decisions about many troublesome aspects of this subject. In spite of organizational and ethical standards, however, many unresolved issues remain. Perhaps this will always be so, since ethical standards change with our ideology, and ideologic changes are continuous.

It has been suggested that investigators stay apprised of societal changes and adjust their practices to insure that they are congruent with those changes. But investigators can do more than that. They can, through their own professional practice, demonstrate and communicate the value of enhancing the quality of human life in every way possible. Two contemporary humanitarians chose the same word, collaboration, to describe how the quality of human life can be enhanced through research.

Katz suggests that subjects be invited to share an adventure in a search for new knowledge instead of being asked to be used as research subjects. He points out that a collaborator in research shares in the highest level of need satisfaction possible, the personal satisfaction of having made a contribution toward the betterment of society. He says if the subject is personally involved through his interest in the problem, his motivation to collaborate in a socially worthwhile endeavor, he will not be suspicious, nor will he feel like a guinea pig.[47]

Mead supports that viewpoint and says that promulgating research as a collaborative effort would have a profound effect on public reaction to research. She then says that, instead of thinking of research as something to be avoided, people might think of it as an opportunity to collaborate in an intellectual adventure, a form of responsible citizenship. Mead believes this viewpoint of research might result in a widespread desire to participate, just as people now donate their bodies and organs to science after their death.[48]

Research, when human rights are meticulously protected, can provide an opportunity for professionals and laymen to work together as collaborators in a search for new knowledge, each contributing in the way in which he is able toward the goal of the betterment of mankind. A collaborative relationship requires complete understanding on both parts. It is incompatible with any kind of exploitation or coercion. It embodies the essence of enhancing human rights and the quality of life and that, after all, is what the protection of human subjects is all about.

REFERENCES

1. H. Beecher, "Experimentation in Man," *JAMA* 169 (January 31, 1959): 461.

2. "New Horizons in Medical Ethics: Research Investigations in Children," *Br Med J* 2 (May 19, 1973): 406.

3. J. Katz, "The Education of the Physician-investigator," in P. Freund (ed.), *Experimentation with Human Subjects* (New York: Braziller, 1969), p. 297.

4. *Ibid.*, p. 295.

5. R. McCormick, "Proxy Consent in the Experimentation Situation," *Perspect. Biol. Med.* 18 (Autumn 1974): 2-20.

6. J. Katz, *Experimentation with Human Beings* (New York: Russell Sage, 1972), p. 855.

7. F. Abdellah, "Approaches to Protecting the Rights of Human Subjects," *Nurs Res* 16 (Fall 1967): 316-20.

8. E. Langer, "Human Experimentation: New York Verdict Affirms Patient's Rights," *Science* 151 (February 11, 1966): 663-66.

9. A. Capron, "Legal Considerations Affecting Clinical Pharmacological Studies in Children," *Clin Res* 21 (February 1973): 141-50.

10. B. Hirsch, "The Medicolegal Framework for Clinical Research in Medicine," *Ann NY Acad Sci* 169 (January–February 1970): 308-15.

11. "Research Projects Involving Human Subjects," *NIH Guide* 3 (August 26, 1974): 1-2, 12.

12. American Nurses' Association, *Human Rights Guidelines for Nurses in Clinical and Other Research,* (Kansas City, Mo.: American Nurses' Association, 1975).

13. R. Alfidi, "Informed Consent: a Study of Patient Reaction," *JAMA* 216 (May 24, 1971): 1325-29.

14. B. Gray, "An Assessment of Institutional Review Committees in Human Experimentation," *Nurs Dig* 4 (Summer 1976): 28-31.

15. "The Two-Part Consent Form," *N Engl J Med* 290 (April 25, 1974): 964-66.

16. O. Ruebhausen and O. Brim, "Privacy and Behavioral Research," *Am Psychol* 21 (May 1966): 423-37.

17. "Privacy Act of 1974," *NIH Guide* 5 (April 28, 1976): 1-4.

18. I. Ladimer, "Protection and Compensation for Injury in Human Studies," in P. Freund (ed.), *Experimentation with Human Subjects* (New York: Braziller, 1969), p. 252.

19. B. Barber, "The Ethics of Experimentation with Human Subjects," *Sci Am* 234 (February 1976): 25-31.

20. L. Altman, "Auto-experimentation: an Unappreciated Tradition in Medical Science," *N Engl J Med* 286 (February 17, 1972): 346-52.

21. D. Martin, "Human Subjects in Clinical Research," *N Engl J Med* 279 (December 26, 1968): 1426-31.

22. J. Katz, *Experimentation with Human Beings* (New York: Russell Sage, 1972), p. 305.

23. C. Lowe, "Pediatrics: Proper Utilization of Children as Research Subjects," *Ann NY Acad Sci* 169 (January–February 1970): 337-43.

24. "New Horizons in Medical Ethics: Research Investigations and the Fetus," *Br Med J* 2 (May 26, 1973): 464–68.

25. W. Curran and H. Beecher, "Experimentation in Children," *JAMA* 210 (October 6, 1969): 77–83.

26. A. Schwartz, "Children's Concepts of Research Hospitalization," *N Engl J Med* 287 (November 21, 1972): 589–92.

27. A. Hofmann and H. Pilpel, "The Legal Rights of Minors," *Pediatr Clin North Am* 20 (November 1973): 989–1004.

28. H. Beecher, "Scarce Resources and Medical Advancement," in P. Freund (ed.), *Experimentation with Human Subjects* (New York: Braziller, 1969), p. 76.

29. D. Mills, "Whither Informed Consent?" *JAMA* 229 (July 15, 1974): 305–10.

30. F. Ayd, "Drug Studies in Prison Volunteers," *South Med J* 65 (April 1972): 440–44.

31. J. Katz, *Experimentation with Human Beings* (New York: Russell Sage, 1972), p. 840.

32. S. Jacobson, "Ethical Issues in Experimentation with Human Subjects," *Nurs Forum* 12: 1 (1973): 58–71.

33. J. Lally and B. Barber, "The Compassionate Physician: Frequency and Social Determinants of Physician-investigator Concern for Human Subjects," *Social Forces* 53 (December 1974): 289–96.

34. H. Beecher, "Ethics and Clinical Research," *N Engl J Med* 274 (June 16, 1966): 1354–60.

35. J. Katz, *Experimentation with Human Beings* (New York: Russell Sage, 1972), p. 855.

36. R. Veatch, "Human Experimentation: the Critical Choices Ahead," *Prism* 2 (July 1974): 58–61+.

37. "New Horizons in Medical Ethics: Research Investigations in Adults," *Br Med J* 2 (April 28, 1973): 220–24.

38. "Human Experimentation," *Med World News* 14 (June 8, 1973): 37–51.

39. J. Katz, *Experimentation with Human Beings* (New York: Russell Sage, 1972), p. 889.

40. American Nurses' Association, *Human Rights Guidelines for Nurses in Clinical and Other Research* (Kansas City, Mo.: American Nurses' Association, 1975), p. 8.

41. M. Batey, "Some Methodological Issues in Research," *Nurs Res* 19 (November–December 1970): 511–16.

42. "Protecting the Rights of Research Subjects," *Nurs Res* 18 (November–December, 1969): 483.

43. "Ethical Considerations in the Publication of the Results of Research Involving Human Subjects," *Clin Res* 21 (October 1973): 763–67.

44. American Nurses' Association, *Human Rights Guidelines for Nurses in Clinical and Other Research* (Kansas City, Mo.: American Nurses' Association, 1975), p. 1.

45. *Ibid.*, p. 3.

46. R. Savard, "Serving Investigator, Patient, and Community in Research Studies," *Ann NY Acad Sci* 169 (January–February 1970): 429–34.

47. J. Katz, *Experimentation with Human Beings* (New York: Russell Sage, 1972), p. 589.

48. M. Mead, "Research with Human Beings: a Model Derived from Anthropological Field Practice," in P. Freund (ed.), *Experimentation with Human Subjects* (New York: Braziller, 1969), p. 164.

CHAPTER SEVEN

THE FUTURE OF NURSING RESEARCH

Juanita W. Fleming

The future of nursing research is uncertain as no one can know the future. A futurologist would however be capable of making some possible predictions about the future in spite of the many and complex issues which confront the nursing profession. This chapter is not concerned with prediction or even necessarily with the many unresolved issues, but rather with some thoughts based on present trends and current issues which may affect nursing research, and which will hopefully provide a perspective on the future for those interested in research. There are few issues in nursing so charged with emotion as those of nursing research.

The profession is composed of a number of subgroups. Some of these are based on clinical practice, e.g., maternal-child nursing; others on functional roles, e.g., nurse administrator; and others on a combination of the two, e.g., teacher of maternal-child nursing. The American Nurses' Association—the professional association of American nurses—probably has the largest nurse membership of any of the professional organizations. However, a large percentage of the almost 1,000,000 registered nurses in this country do not belong to the association. Consequently, on many of the issues in nursing the response of nurses seems to reflect the individualism of the groups rather than the collective response of the profession as a whole. The significance of the subgroups in nursing and the professional association is that they have some choice in affecting the future of nursing research.

ACCEPTANCE OF RESEARCH IN NURSING

Research in nursing, unlike many other issues, appears to be one which professional nurses accept as an important and legitimate activity in the profession regardless of group affiliation. This is not to say that there are not diverse opinions about research among nurses. Three distinct views are expressed by Jacox, Hayes and Notter. Notter sees nursing research as every nurse's business,[1] while Hayes clearly states that nursing research is not every nurse's business.[2] Jacox's view is that "nursing can never develop a scientific basis for its practice until practitioners themselves—not just the "career" researchers—have a great deal more involvement in research."[3]

Nursing research, like all research, is viewed as the creation or production of knowledge. The goal of nursing research is to enlarge the body of knowledge which will enable the profession to meet its commitment to society though the work of its professionals. Nurses in general seem to accept this premise.

Some of the indicators that suggest that research in nursing is an activity accepted by nurses are as follows.

(1) The number of articles about research that appear in nursing publications. Many articles in nursing publications are not only about nursing research but often actually publish research findings. The case for nursing research is presently more evident than in the past. This is likely so because there is an acceptance that nursing has a distinctive professional service to offer. Notter says, "Obviously, if nursing has a distinctive service to offer, then researchable questions about how to improve that service can be asked. Thus, a body of knowledge that underlies practice can be developed."[4]

(2) The establishment in 1952 of the refereed journal *Nursing Research*. The number of subscription holders of this journal in comparison to others published by the American Journal of Nursing Company is small. However, nurses generally seem to agree that this is a worthwhile publication and that the expectation of large numbers of subscriptions should not be its reason for existence. Many nurse scholars view the publication as essential to the profession.

(3) The publishing of another refereed journal in nursing entitled *Research in Nursing and Health*. This journal invites manuscripts which report original research in the areas of nursing practice, education and administration; health issues relevant to nursing; and investigations of implementation of research findings in clinical settings.

(4) The designation of a structural unit—The Commission on Nursing Research—in the American Nurses' Association (ANA) which specifically considers issues related to nursing research. The Commission consists of elected and appointed members of the ANA. These individuals are accountable

for developing and implementing a program of activity to advance nursing research.

(5) The establishment of the Council of Nurse Researchers within the American Nurses' Association. This group is composed of members and associate members of the American Nurses' Association who have earned master's or higher degrees, are engaged in the conduct of research or in guiding students and/or registered nurses in research, or are serving as consultants in research. The Council's purpose is to advance research activities, to provide for the exchange of ideas, and to recognize excellence in research.

(6) The increased number of positions for nurse researchers in hospitals and educational institutions. Nurse researchers are being hired for the purpose of promoting and enhancing research of nurses in hospitals and educational environs. There is growing recognition that nurses with research training are prepared to conduct independent studies and/or assume the role of facilitator of research.

(7) The inclusion of research content in the basic professional curricula and master's programs accredited by the National League for Nursing. A practice orientation is frequently emphasized at both the baccalaureate and master's levels. The pattern seems to be a much heavier emphasis on practice at the baccalaureate level, with a very small portion on research. At the master's level clinical fields of study and preparation of a functional area are emphasized. Research content is included in most master's programs and students enrolled in these programs often complete a thesis or a systematic inquiry project of some sort. Based on the way the educational programs are organized, it seems that the positions of Notter, Hayes, and Jacox can each be defended. All nurses should at least have an appreciation for the essence of nursing research, and the inclusion of some research in the basic program is therefore necessary. The need for master's-prepared clinicians to involve themselves in research seems essential if research in nursing is to move forward. Thus the research content included in the master's program is designed not to prepare a researcher but to develop beginning skills in this direction.

(8) The establishment of doctoral programs designed to prepare nurse researchers and the increased number of nurses entering doctoral programs. Unlike the baccalaureate and master's degrees in nursing, the doctoral degree program for researchers is basically research-oriented. The need for rigorously trained researchers in nursing is absolutely essential if sound research is to be produced.

The nurse researcher has to be cognizant of the difference between what is researchable and what compromises can be made by scientific rigor and within the confines of good research. Inadequate skill in and knowledge of research principles and research methods lead to an unhealthy reliance on specific techniques that are used whether or not they are the most adequate for a given purpose.[2]

The development of competent nurse researchers is seen as essential to the profession. In doctoral study, students have an opportunity to work with faculty members who are productive researchers. They learn to differentiate between fields of practice (e.g., maternity, pediatrics, medical-surgical, etc.) and intellectual problems of nursing research. Students' abilities to carry out the research process are strengthened through courses in methodology and statistics and through opportunities to engage in research activities.

(9) The increased number of research conferences and meetings which focus on research. Examples are the Eastern Research Conference and the Western Research Conference. Meetings to share research results and discuss research problems are held at various universities throughout the country.

Further evidence of the acceptance of nursing research as a legitimate activity is found in the responses of government and private organizations. A few follow.

(a) Sigma Theta Tau, National Honor Society of Nursing—emphasis on nursing research. In keeping with the purposes of recognition of scholarship of superior quality and encouragement of creative work, research is the natural focus of this organization. Funds to support research are awarded by the organization on a competitive basis.

(b) The minority nurse research fellowship program of the American Nurses' Association, supported with funds from the National Institute of Mental Health. This program is designed to increase the number of minority group nurses with doctorates. The nurses enroll in programs throughout the United States and pursue various aspects of the profession.

(c) Nursing Research Grants, designed to support basic and clinical research, are available through the United States Department of Health, Education, and Welfare, Public Health Manpower, Division of Nursing. The program supports research related to the care process, and seeks to enlarge institutional nursing research capabilities, foster scientific communication, and address significant questions in nursing education, manpower, and administration.

The same agency administers a pre- and post-doctoral nurse fellowship program. The purposes of this program, which gives the National Research Service Awards authorized under Public Law 94-278, Title II, are to increase the opportunities for qualified nurses to engage in full-time graduate and research training; to prepare professional nurses to conduct independent research, collaborate in interdisciplinary research, and stimulate and guide others in nursing research; to promote the availability and utilization of nurses with research training in nursing and/or the basic sciences as faculty in schools of nursing at undergraduate and graduate levels; and to prepare nurses to conduct scientific inquiry in disciplines that have significance for nursing theory and practice.[5]

An acceptance of the status of research in our society is another issue. An optimism about the future and a sense that progress was inevitable pervaded American society during the early 1900s. This optimism has stayed with us to some extent, although there have been cycles of good and bad times. However, in spite of certain setbacks there are now such positive indicators as increased affluence, improved technology, etc. Research in nursing seems to have followed this trend. It too has had its up and down periods. In spite of the down periods it persists as an essential component of the nursing profession. Support of nursing research, however, is not stable and may never be stable (support for most other research is also unstable). The concerns regarding support can be divided into four main categories: dependability of funding for research, vitality of the research system, freedom within the research system, and public confidence in science and technology.[6] These concerns are elaborated on elsewhere in this chapter.

SCOPE OF NURSING RESEARCH

Trying to distinguish between nursing research and research in nursing poses an interesting problem. Gortner distinguishes between the two as follows

> The first has as its subject the care process and the problems that are encountered in the practice of nursing: maintenance of hygiene, rest, sleep, nutrition, relief from pain or discomfort, counseling, health education, and rehabilitation. The second has as its subject the profession itself,[7] its practitioners and the characteristics of their practices: utilization, costs, administration, career patterns, educational level of nurses and nurse students.

Abdellah further states:

> Nursing research is a systematic detailed attempt to discover or confirm facts that relate to a specific problem or problems in nursing. . . . When the ultimate goal is the application of scientific knowledge to improve nursing practice, this is referred to as clinical research in nursing.[8]

The Commission of Nursing Research gave the following statement about nursing research.

Research in nursing addresses the human and behavioral questions that arise in the treatment of disease and the prevention of illness and maintenance of health. Some of the human questions that must be answered are:

How are individuals helped to maintain health?

How are individuals persuaded to use available measures to prevent illness?

How are people helped to cope with illness when it comes?

How are complications for hospitalized or chronically ill people reduced?

How is illness prevented for people who are highly subject to health risks such as premature infants and the elderly?[9]

Leininger believes that nursing and health care phenomena will be explored vigorously during the next decade. She states, "The essence of health service lies with caring support behaviors and caring activities . . . all of which is the heart of nursing."[10] She notes that the art and science of nursing care—caring cultures, caring processes, and caring outcomes—have hardly been tapped by nurse researchers.

It is safe to conclude that there are many definitions of nursing research. There are also many views regarding individual preparation and involvement. There is growing recognition that research is necessary for continued growth and improvement of the nursing profession. Nurses, like other health professionals, work cooperatively to serve those who need health care. They carry out surveillance of health for individuals in all states of wellness and illness. They provide sustaining and supportive services to those with whom they work, either to restore them to optimal health or to help them have a peaceful death. Nurse scholars now recognize the need for growth of the scientific body of knowledge in nursing. The science of nursing can be defined as the critical body of knowledge arrived at through research and logical analysis.

The scope and focus of nursing practice are broad and so, consequently, is the scope of nursing research. In consideration of the future of nursing research, some potentially promising areas for research will now be presented.

Research Priorities

Basic scientific research has lost some of its funding recently. Abelson remarks, "At one time basic research was comparatively well supported . . . of late, however, there has been a sharp decrease in long-term support for fundamental work. Instead, much of the effort . . . is now devoted to quick payoff activities, such as improving existing products and cutting costs."[6]

The cost of health care services is exorbitant. Research which will aid in minimizing the cost of services, yet still allow quality care, is an area in which nurse researchers could assume an aggressive course of action. The need for basic research in nursing certainly exists now, and small amounts will continue to be done. However, much of the research in nursing falls into the category of applied research, and this is likely to continue.

Nursing does not exist in a vacuum and consequently, as with other health professions, its members must consider the future health care needs of the American people. This is essential because nurses have and will continue to have an essential role in meeting the health care needs of our society. There seems to be a "quality of life" research. Senator Kennedy noted, in his 1976 Washington Report on Health Legislation, "We have demonstrated our capacity to do basic research. However, we will not have fulfilled our contract with the taxpayers until we have matched the excellence of our efforts in basic research with a comparable effort to apply new knowledge to improve the quality of day to day health care in every community in our nation."

Applied research in nursing by definition deals with existing problems concerning life situations and basic recognized needs. There are many health care problems to which nurse researchers can contribute. Setting priorities in nursing research can be viewed as undesirable, but there are pressing problems in the world which could benefit from immediate research. For example, infectious diseases and malnutrition plague millions of children in various parts of the world. To ignore this and other problems would be inhumane. Priorities for clinical nursing research could be viewed as helpful guidelines.[11] Further, a priority statement could be employed to interpret the significance of certain programs of research as well as to indicate the general scope of nursing.

The scope and focus of nursing have not been publicized as well as with some other health care professions. Nursing practice, education, and research all focus on determining the health status and maximizing the health potential of each person served with scientifically sound, humanistic nursing care.[12]

Holistic Approach to Health Care

Salk, discoverer of the polio vaccine, told a large medical audience that mankind is entering a new epoch in which holistic medicine will be the dominant model. He views the future in terms of health, which he defines as a properly functioning whole. In the future, according to Salk, mankind will use cooperation rather than competition, influence rather than power, tools rather than weapons, birth control rather than death control. He sees the holistic health movement as inevitable, and from a life-affirming perspective emerging with the new epoch.[13]

The holistic approach to health is a concept espoused by nurses. Human beings are seen as more than and different from the sum of their parts. The basic assumptions, by Roger's definition, on which nursing science builds are as follows.

1. Man is a unified whole, possessing his own integrity and manifesting characteristics that are more than and different from the sum of his parts.
2. Man and environment are continuously exchanging matter and energy with one another.
3. The life process evolves irreversibly and unidirectionally along the space-time continuum.
4. Pattern and organization identify man and reflect his innovative wholeness.
5. Man is characterized by the capacity for abstraction and imagery, language and thought, sensation and emotion.[14]

RESEARCH NEEDS

Preventive Health

The core of modern health care is not only illness prevention that can reduce mortality and mobidity but the very special kind of prevention that flows from self-help. Ubell explains this issue as follows.

> Treatment of disease may very well have reached the limit of its effectiveness in controlling disease in populations. . . . It is becoming clearer that what individuals in our society do with their bodies from early childhood onward is more controlling over health over the long span of years than anything physicians and disease care technicians can do for them once they are ill.[15]

Ubell further declares that George Bernard Shaw recognized long ago that the social and psychological environment probably contributes more to health than medicine and medicators.

A recognition that medical care is only one aspect of the broader field of health seems to be somewhat prevalent. A rethinking of the role of society, the institutions in society, and the individual in preventive health is necessary. Early preventive health starting in childhood can achieve gains in lifetime health status and play an important role in formulating long-term attitudes toward health.[16] Individuals must somehow recognize that neither the physician nor other health care workers can be expected to overcome the consequences of a lifetime of health-damaging behavior. Breslow and Somers propose a lifetime health monitoring program.[17] Their practical approach to preventive medicine uses clinical and epidemiological criteria to identify the specific health goals and professional services appropriate to ten different age groups, from infancy to 75 years and over. They suggest that the cost of this type of preventive care be covered by health insurance plans based on fee-for-service or capitation.

The area of preventive health involves the actions of many people. A need to understand man's health-seeking behavior is important. There are a great number of behaviors which are detrimental to health and increase the risk of ill health. A few of these are: excess use of alcohol and mood-altering drugs; cigarette smoking; poor nutritional practices; carelessness, which results in injuries caused by accidents; sedentary lifestyles and improper exercise; and improper care and supervision of children by indolent parents, or by those who lack the proper knowledge to carry out a parenting role.

One approach to the study of future preventable health problems in nursing is to consider the age continuum. Preventive health problems are a concern for all age groups. However, the two extreme age groups each present unique problems.

The Young

Ziegler noted that an estimated two-thirds of our nation's 6.6 million children receive inadequate medical attention and an additional 25 million receive little more than marginal care. A survey revealed that millions of children are not protected against polio (15.5 million), diptheria (9.3 million), measles (13.8 million), rubella (13.9 million), or mumps (26.4 million).[18] In spite of the success in the control and prevention of these diseases, the immunization levels among children in this country are unacceptably low.

According to Mullen the "state of the child" report done by the Foundation of Child Development presents statistics which reflect the poor quality of life of children in New York City. He states that "A review of national statistics suggests that the fundamental experiences of New York city's children are not unlike those of the rest of the nation's approximately 80 million youngsters."[19] This seems to suggest that parents need help with the care of their children. The parenting role in a highly complex society is probably much more difficult and is likely to become even more so. Other problems which focus on parent-child relationships, such as negligence and abuse, are also concerns.

HEW's *Forward Plan for Health* states, "The number of children under fifteen in mental institutions more than doubled between 1955 and 1973."[16] Further research to prevent psychosocial disability is likely to gain support. The research discovery of bonding between mother and infant immediately after birth correlated with improved health and psychosocial functioning of the child. This was a relatively simple intervention program which was cost effective. The need to implement cost effective intervention programs which will improve the quality of life for children and their families is essential. The 1978-1982 Child Health Preventive Plan focuses on five problem areas requiring special attention: (1) decreasing the incidence of disabling conditions; (2) decreasing the rate and adverse consequences of teenage pregnancies; (3) raising immunization levels to protect children against childhood diseases; (4) increasing preventive mental health services to families and youth; and (5) providing health education to improve access to comprehensive care.[16]

The Aged

Woodruff predicts that by the year 2020 thirteen percent of the United States' population will be over 65 years of age.[20] The aged have a unique set of problems and finding the best solutions to these problems is likely to require considerable study. The 1971 White House Conference on Aging emphasized the need for immediate and special consideration of problems and services for the aged.

The American population may simply be getting older. The statistics on births seem to show that fewer and fewer babies are being born and that the life expectancies of males and females are on the increase. The future population of America is likely to contain a considerably greater percentage of older people. Demographers are observing the rate of change in the composition of the population. It follows logically that if more individuals are living longer and fewer are being born each year the demographic balance will be perceptibly altered. The changes which will result in the society as the population becomes older may be viewed by some as negative and others as positive. The question for nurse researchers is: how will this change affect nursing? The fact that the number of children seems destined to decrease, as the aged population increases, is likely to have a profound effect on nursing education as well as nursing service. The economics of maintaining and caring for the aged, and the need to consider the aspects of leisure time, retirement, coping abilities, health status, and socioeconomic status are all important factors which might be studied. If there are few children, will there be more child-centered homes? Will a higher premium be placed on the young? Based on the information available, one could conclude as follows.

(1) The population growth rate is declining primarily because of the dramatic drop in birth rates. The decline in fertility rates will likely affect the health care system in the following ways: (a) decreased demand for hospital obstetric units; (b) decreased demand for hospital pediatric units, partially because of low fertility but also because of advances reducing the need to hospitalize children; (c) reduction of neonatal mortality because of better contraception and greater ease of obtaining abortions; and (d) tendency of the population to be older because fewer babies are being born and people are living longer. Several factors seem to contribute to a longer life: better health care, higher standard of living, and new medical discoveries.[21]

(2) The demand for health care will be essentially from the aged. This group has more health problems and consequently requires more health care. When a patient is hospitalized, the stay will likely be longer. For all conditions requiring hospitalization, the average length of stay for older people is 12.6 days, as contrasted with 5.7 days for patients between 15 and 44 and 4.7 days for those under 15.[22]

A second approach to the study of future research problems in nursing is to consider types of care, e.g., primary health care and long-term health care. Judging from present nursing concerns, both primary and long-term care are areas of focus.

Primary Health Care

There is some controversy regarding primary health care, which does not seem to be so with long-term health care. Grace pointed out the need to speak in a definitive way on the nature of primary nursing. She noted—in her commentary on the proceedings of the scientific session of the American Academy of Nursing—the need to be clearer regarding the role of the nurse who is practicing primary care.[23]

The researchable questions regarding primary health care are multiple. Chances are that improved health care services will be implemented for the entire population, regardless of socioeconomic status. Changes in the delivery system would then be necessary. Instead of large numbers of hospitals delivering care, there are likely to be primary care centers with health managers, which are more accessible to the people to be served. The question of how best to plan, deliver, assess, and monitor care for all age and socioeconomic groups, along with a variety of other questions, can be generated in the area of primary health care. The entire area of assessment of health lends itself to study.

Long-Term Health Care

The multitude of problems which evolve from long-term illness presents an unusual challenge to nurse researchers. Nurse leaders have recognized this as a present and future problem in which nursing input is essential. There are varied conditions and concerns with which individuals with chronic health problems and their families have to cope.

The American Academy of Nursing has recognized as one of its challenges the need "to identify and propose resolutions to issues and problems confronting nursing and health, including alternative plans for implementation." At the 1976 annual meeting the scientific session dealt with long-term care. A publication entitled *Long-Term Care in Perspective: Past, Present and Future Directions for Nursing* resulted.[24]

It follows logically that if our society has an increase in its percentage of older people it is likely to have an increase in long-term illness. Although many older people are healthy, many also suffer from one or more chronic conditions. The conditions which are most often seen include diabetes, urological conditions, arthritis, cardiac conditions, glaucoma, cataracts, cancer, and cerebral vascular accidents. Mental aberrations affect some of the aged and result in varied behavior which may often lead to misdiagnosis.

The incidence of major cardiovascular diseases in the United States continues to be a serious problem. The estimated number of people afflicted with heart diseases, high blood pressure, strokes, arteriosclerosis, etc., was 28.4 million.[25] The number of people being treated for mental illness is also growing. In 1955 there were 1,675,000 people under treatment for mental illness. By 1971 the figure was 4,038,000.[25]

One approach to future researchable problems in nursing is to consider particular conditions which are now prevalent and are likely to be prevalent in the future. Drug abuse is an example of this type of problem.

Drug Abuse

Excess use of drugs and problems associated with drug abuse present a multiplicity of researchable problems. Drug addiction is on the increase. The number of new narcotic addicts rose from 6,012 in 1965 to 24,692 in 1972.[26] The age group of people between 18 and 20 has the largest proportion of individuals who have experienced a problem associated with drinking. One out of seven high school males (14 percent) report getting drunk at least once per week.[27]

The effect of drugs taken by the mother on unborn babies is believed by some to be deleterious, particularly with heroin, methadone, and alcohol. The high incidence of prematurity and the incidence of complications among infants of heroin-addicted and methadone-maintained mothers (IHMM) has been well documented.[28]

Untoward effects of alcohol and cigarette smoking on the fetus are highly suspected. Fetal alcohol syndrome may result from excessive use of alcohol by pregnant women. The effect of cigarette smoking on the unborn infant is uncertain but thought to be deleterious. Little is known regarding the long-term effects of these drugs on infant growth and development. Presumably, the infant whose mother uses drugs during pregnancy experiences an alteration of his predetermined growth channel while in utero. The frequency of prematurity seems to substantiate this. Further deviations from the already altered channel of growth may take place during the withdrawal period, which is manifested through the central nervous system, the gastrointestinal system, and the respiratory system.[29]

The study of addicted individuals continues to pose challenging problems for researchers in many disciplines, including nursing. It is believed by some in our society that habitual drug use enables the user to cope with daily living. As our society becomes more complex and impersonal, the use of drugs is likely to increase if other more healthy means for coping are not established. The drug orientation which seems to be prevalent in our society creates an environment in which the use of all types of drugs, including mood-altering drugs, tends to be more acceptable.

Stress

In a society which appears to be rapidly changing and in which those who are to survive adequately must be able to adjust quickly, a high level of stress results. The increased incidence of psychological and psychiatric problems seems evident. Many illnesses of the future will no doubt be directly associated with stress. In order for our society to remain viable, change is absolutely necessary. Change creates stress. More knowledge of how stress affects individuals is essential. Selye, in his popular *Stress of Life,* provided much light on what stress does to the human condition. Stress management will become an important aspect of the therapeutic approach in helping people cope with health problems. Identifying, assessing, measuring, and implementing intervention plans to alter loneliness, pain, fear, and other precursors of adjustment problems in people of all ages provide a real challenge for the nurse scientist.

Venereal Disease

The incidence of venereal disease is thought to have reached epidemic proportions. The accuracy of the statistics are questionable and the incidence may even be higher. The known statistics reflect only those reported to the National Center for Disease Control in Atlanta, Georgia.

Cancer

The incidence of cancer is high, particularly among blacks, women, and children of ages 3 to 14. Development of behaviors which will enable the individuals with cancer and their families to cope is an important area of study in cancer research. Research is needed on patients' psychological responses to particular types of treatment, along with research on the best physical treatment or cure of the disease.

Nutrition Problems

Nutrition problems are widespread in America, ranging from undernutrition to obesity in all age groups; and involving the quality and safety of food. Adequate food and sound nutrition is essential for human survival and are prerequisites for improving the quality of life.

These conditions and many others which have not been mentioned are potential areas of nursing research.

Cultural Diversity

Our society is a blend of many subcultures. Unfortunately, this diversity is often viewed more as a problem than as a resource for helping to solve health problems. Research which will facilitate our understanding of the health behaviors associated with different cultures seems desirable. Behaviors of persons from other cultures and the various subcultures in our own society are all too often misunderstood and unaccepted.

Problems Identified by Nurses

Another approach to future researchable problems in nursing is to consider those which nurses have identified as appropriate and needing to be studied.

Individual nurses' interest in the practice areas of research is evident in the nursing literature. For example, Williams[30] believes it is important to investigate the characteristics of nurse practitioners and their educational programs, but urges that characteristics of the practice setting should also be investigated. Ketefian's[31] concern, regarding the application of research in practice, is well illustrated in a pilot study describing the utilization of a research finding on temperatures by nurses. Gortner and colleagues[32] point out the contributions of nursing research in patient care. Studies are identified which contribute to modern practice and/or seem oriented toward the future.

Lindeman[11] reports that a panel of nurses who participated in a nationwide survey identified 15 of the most important areas of research for the profession. These were as follows.

1. Determination of means for greater utilization of research in practice.
2. Determination of valid and reliable indicators of quality nursing care.
3. Establishment of the relationship between clinical nursing research and quality care.
4. Evaluation of the effects of expanding the role of the nurse in patient care, and clarification of this concept.
5. Delimitation and evalution of the functions and clinical parameters of independent nurse practitioners.
6. Development of a set of physical and psychological assessment procedures that provides information necessary for nursing intervention and improved patient care.
7. Determination and evaluation of interventions by nurses that are most effective in reducing psychological stress of patients.
8. Evaluation, in terms of patient outcomes, of processes used to provide nursing care.
9. Determination of valid, reliable methods for establishing nursing staffing patterns that adequately reflect patient needs and cost containment.
10. Evaluation, in terms of patient outcomes, of the role of the nurse in preventive health services.
11. Assessment of the relationship between the quality of nursing leadership and the quality of nursing practice in institutions.
12. Evaluation of the effectiveness of various approaches to peer review.
13. Exploration of means of enhancing nurses' ability to cope with stress when working in high-stress environments.
14. Determination of effective means of communicating, evaluating, and implementing change in practice.
15. Determination of the nursing behaviors and settings for care most likely to produce positive effects on an individual or family in a (health) crisis-prone situation.

In 1975 the American Nurses' Association Commission on Nursing Research published a paper entitled *Priorities for Research in Nursing, 1975*. The Commission's priorities for research were divided into two categories: questions related to the practice of nursing and questions related to the profession of nursing. Some of the studies identified for practice are: studies to reduce complications of hospitalization and surgery (sleep deprivation, anorexia, diarrhea, neurosensory disturbance, respiratory infections, circulatory problems, etc.); studies to improve the outlook for high-risk parents and high-risk infants; studies to improve the health care of the elderly; studies of life-threatening situations, anxiety, pain, and stress; studies of adaptation to chronic illness and the development of self care systems; studies to facilitate the successful utilization of new technological developments in patient care; studies of nursing intervention to promote health; studies to facilitate the successful application of new knowledge to patient care; studies to define and delineate healthy states; studies of addictive and adherence behaviors; studies of undernutrition and overnutrition; and studies to evaluate the outcomes and/or effectiveness to consumers and providers of different patterns of delivery of nursing services. The six studies identified by the Commission pertaining to the profession of nursing are: (1) studies of manpower for nursing education, practice, and research; (2) studies of quality assurance for nursing and of criterion measures for practice and education; (3) studies of cost-effectiveness of nursing utilization and preparation in relation to acute care, long-term care, extended care, and community health; (4) studies in the history and philosophy of nursing; (5) studies in nursing curricula; and (6) studies in the organization of the nursing profession.[33]

Environmental Concerns

A final approach which may be considered in identifying researchable problems in nursing concerns the environment. Our highly industrialized nation faces environmental problems which may be classified as psycho-social problems or problems of the physical environment. The psycho-social problems are those brought about by stress, which leads to high incidences of mental disease, suicide, and crime. The alienation of people from one another because of high mobility necessitates their having to establish many new relationships—most of which will be temporary or fleeting. The rapidity and constancy with which individuals must adjust to change may be a major source of stress. The constancy in which change and the establishment of new relationships for survival occur creates an instability which may affect health status.

The effects of pollution—air, water, and noise—on the health of individuals certainly needs more research. We need to know how to control or minimize pollution and still maintain or increase affluence.

Finally, the utilization and distribution of world resources and consequent effects on developing nations, as well as on such highly industrialized societies as our own, should be viewed from an environmental perspective.

There is certainly no dearth of problems for research in which nurses can engage now and in the future. Many of the findings on problems for which studies can be formulated may also help solve other problems. Inquiry into the nature of humans and the conditions in which they find themselves engenders unique problems not always easy to specify. Nursing research or research in nursing, depending on the nature of the problems studied, offers a challenge for the future which is unprecedented.

Many problem areas have been identified in which research could improve the quality of life. Ways to prepare to meet this challenge are presented in the final section of this chapter.

POLITICAL ACTION

Nurse scientists, like all scientists, need to become more politically astute. This necessitates becoming acquainted with social and political processes. The profession of nursing has the makings of a powerful force if some agreement on action can be collectively made. Recognition of what the society needs and wants is basic to political action.

Health related research is all systematic study directed toward the development and use of scientific knowledge in the following areas:

1. The causes, diagnosis, treatment, control, prevention of, and rehabilitation relating to, the physical and mental diseases and other killing and crippling impairments of mankind;
2. The origin nature and solution of health problems not identifiable in terms of disease entities;
3. Broad fields of science important to or underlying disease and health problems; and
4. Research in nutritional problems impairing, contributing to, or otherwise affecting optimal health; and all research performed by an organization whose primary mission is health oriented.[34]

The statement above appeared in a report of the 87th Congress, in 1961, in a chapter entitled "Health Research—A National Resource." The chapter began, "Research might be regarded as one of the two main supports on which the health of the nation rests." This may be viewed as rhetoric by some, but it seems to be a basic truth from which researchers interested in the health of the people of this country can take heart. Though there is no law which states an overall health goal, in the preamble to the comprehensive Health Planning and Public Health Service Amendments (1966), Congress does declare that fulfillment of our national purpose depends on promoting and assuring the highest level of health attainable for every person, in an environment which contributes positively to healthful individual and family living.

Society's acceptance that health care is a right for all, rather than a privilege, creates new or at least additional roles for health professionals. The value of a healthy population for our national security and well-being is as political today as it was in 1961. This is evident by the pieces of legislation which have provisions for health care for various population groups in American society. More than 75 pieces of health legislation have been passed since 1961. Examples are the Migrant Health Act, which authorizes federal aid for clinics; the Family Planning and Population Research Act, which is the largest single source of public funds supporting family planning services, and the Cost Containment Act. Legislation specific to mentally retarded individuals, and to people with such conditions as sickle cell anemia, Cooley's anemia, and diabetes, is indicative of the provisions enacted for particular groups. The Noise Control Act, the Clean Water Act, and the Clean Air Act are for environmental health. Medicare, a health insurance program for the aged; Medicaid, a state-operated program designed to help defray the health care costs of the poor and medically indigent; and the health maintenance Organization Act, which assisted in establishing and expanding health maintenance organizations (HMOs), are other examples of legislation for specific segments of the population.

Quality assurance programs have demanded much attention. The cost of health care and other factors have given rise to professional standards review organizations (PSROs). The organizations are to monitor the adequacy of and necessity for care given to patients in health care institutions. The improvement of the quality of care given in institutions, and the push toward a national health insurance (which seems imminent), reflect the values of American society; that is, that a healthy population is most desirable.

An awareness of trends which are likely to have a political impact is essential for nurse scientists. For example, more of the population of the United States is likely to live in urban communities than in rural and small town communities in the future. In addition, technological advances are changing the health care system. Two types of technological changes that affect, and are likely to continue to affect, care systems are administrative technology— which is related to data processing, telemonitoring, multiphasic screening, and computer work, to aid in operating a more efficient health care system—and clinical technology, which is related to more efficient techniques for identifying, diagnosing and treating health phenomena.

Nurse scientists need to identify scientists in other professions with whom they can cooperate politically to achieve the fundamental goal of nursing research. This writer believes that goal is to answer the human and behavioral questions that arise in the treatment of disease and the prevention of illness, and the maintenance of health.

Reiteration of the importance of research in enhancing the quality of life and in the continuing progress of the country must be made by nurse scientists as well as other scientists. It is suspected that socioeconomic status, cultural background, family background, and home setting contribute to or affect the symptoms and the condition of individuals. These may operate as positive factors in ameliorating health problems or as a negative factor in increasing pathological effects. Scientists working together can identify the combination of factors which enhance health. This country cannot afford to not support research activities. Letters and visits to local and national politicians are essential. However, these activities should be well planned and coordinated. Haphazard handling of these activities may result in more harm than help. Publicity in terms of the contributions of research to the public and as regards those responsible for allocating funds for research must continue. The cultivation of friends of research—particularly the type of research in which nurses wish to engage—may be difficult but is not impossible.

There are a number of professions concerned with aspects of health. Each has a particular role function for which it is accountable. All are concerned with working out methods and means which will lead to the promotion of health and the prevention of disability and infirmity. The roles are expanding as knowledge and technology advance. Though each group of health professionals make decisions unilaterally about the role that group will play in society, it seems that more cooperation among groups is essential. The consumers need to know what they can expect and from whom in the way of health services.

Consumers are a group which nurse scientists need to approach. The average consumer is not as cognizant of nursing research as he could be. An informed, motivated consumer can be a viable political force. The most potent examples of consumer groups in politics are those who worked for the diabetes act, and the parents of trainable retarded children who worked for the legislation that resulted in public education for their children. The future of nursing research holds great promise if nurse scientists can get consumer groups to work for more than an illness-oriented society.

A cost-effective and health-effective program for preventive measures would be desirable. Too few consumers know the extent to which nurses contribute to health care. Every opportunity should be taken to help consumers enhance their knowledge of nursing and nursing research. An informed consumer can be a persuasive advocate for nursing activities.

It does not appear to be politically expedient in our society to ignore those who are capable of making contributions. Consequently, nurse scientists, like other scientists, will be allowed to make contributions if they have worthwhile ones to make. As nurse scientists demonstrate their abilities to contribute they will be accorded more and more opportunities. The expression that nothing succeeds like success is certainly appropriate there. Research that is done well and which makes a contribution is likely to have a positive effect on those responsible for funding research activities.

Industrial research is devoted to more applied or "quick payoff" research. Relationships with industrial companies seem politically wise for nurse scientists from several perspectives. An industry may be a source of funding for research. It may also facilitate the marketing of products produced by nurse-researchers. The future relationship of nurse scientists and the industrial community has tremendous potential.

Though there are countless examples of nursing involvement in the political arena, there are those who take the position that nursing is generally naive when it comes to political action and that this naiveté is reflected in the area of nursing research. There is no advantage in arguing the point. It is, however, important to reiterate the need for nurse scientists to become more politically astute. If scientists, however, have to spend most of their time engaging in political activity, then research will not be done. It therefore would be desirable to develop more effective lobbies for nursing research.

PREPARATION FOR NURSING RESEARCH

In order to be prepared to meet the challenge of the future, nurse scientists must be able to carry out independent research studies. Downs notes that "adequate preparation of doctoral candidates is among the most important and pressing educational issues facing nursing today; for it is upon this core of individuals that we must depend for the critical and creative study of the science of nursing, its theories, and their testing.[35] The need for nurse researchers cannot be overstated. Andreoli noted that much of the research produced in nursing over the past 10 to 15 years was done as a part of the requirement for the master's or doctoral degree.[36] It is obvious that we need more nurses who are prepared to conduct research and who have a commitment to scholarship and the opportunity to produce research beyond their educational programs. The background of investigators is certainly a major factor. However, nursing cannot afford to excuse its lack of contribution to the percentage of female Ph.D.s who for various reasons are unable to conduct research. Nor can we continue to talk about the youth of our profession and the lack of support for research. We must face these issues realistically and seek solutions.

If nursing is to develop doctorally-prepared nurses capable of conducting research, it is essential that certain factors be considered. Some of these are the knowledge base, faculty, administration, students, and resources of the university. Doctoral study in nursing should not be technique, but rather a unified body of facts, concepts, and propositions. The boundaries of knowledge in the discipline of nursing should be further developed and enlarged. The mission of research and doctoral programs designed to produce nurse researchers should be to expand the base of knowledge.

Conceptual frameworks in nursing are developed on a basic commitment to relate scientific and clinical data to the total person, and to identify the additional knowledge needed to make fundamental decisions about that person. The need to develop a more effective communication system among nurses actively engaged in the pursuit of knowledge is essential if theory building is to be facilitated in the profession. Downs has stated as follows.

It is essential in either planning for or trying to maintain a doctoral program that the faculty assess their resources, both personal and financial, in terms of the number of students they believe they can contain within that program. A simple head count of the number of faculty holding doctoral degrees will not yield a satisfactory answer. Even among faculty who hold doctoral degrees, there is considerable variation in their desire for research involvement and their expertise in the process of research. Many, if not most, will lack experience in research beyond their own dissertation. The rigor of the requirements for the degree taken by some of the faculty may differ widely in terms of the research content and the supervision they receive while pursuing the degree. Further, it is a mistake to believe that directing students in an area of inquiry is the same as teaching them in an area of content. There are gross differences between teaching what is known and supporting a candidate through the process of trying to find an answer to what is not known.[35]

The administration and organization of educational units to prepare nurse researchers is critical to the success of the preparation of competent scholars. Recognition that the doctorate is an important step in preparation for scholarly research is essential. The ideals of learning should pervade the atmosphere of the educational unit preparing doctoral students. The student-faculty ratio is important. The quality and quantity of time that the student's sponsor or advisor is able to spend with the student during the dissertation phase of study is critical, since it is during this phase that much of the student's intellectual growth takes place.

In identifying future directions for research, Grace[37] notes that a systematic examination of the process of doctoral education in nursing is essential, along with the resultant productivity and the contributions to patient care. Areas for further exploration include the following.

1. Field tests of institutional collaborative models for offering doctoral education in nursing.
2. Longitudinal studies on graduates from doctoral programs in nursing, in terms of career patterns and impact on nursing education and health care delivery.
3. Evaluation of the effectiveness of different approaches for combining patient care and nursing research activities, both as a doctoral student and as a postdoctoral professional.
4. Comparative studies on the similarities and differences in the competencies of nurses prepared in doctoral programs in nursing, with emphasis on advanced clinical practice and research, and on research and theory development.
5. Studies on the effectiveness of different approaches in increasing the research productivity of nurses with doctorates.
6. Descriptive studies on models for articulating the research programs of faculty members with research interests, as well as the projects of doctoral students.

Research preparation at the doctoral level in nursing, unlike other fields, has not always been evident by the academic degree obtained. Pitel and Vian found a continuing trend whereby nurses are earning the Ph.D. rather than the Ed.D. In the 1950s the Ed.D. was the major type of doctoral degree granted to nurses—over 60% of nurse doctorates were Ed.D.s. In the 1960s the Ph.D. gained ascendancy and this trend continues.

The trend of awarding the Ph.D. degree—the academic or research degree—over the Doctor of Nursing Science (DNS) degree—the professional degree—continued to gain momentum into the 1970s. Predictably, as the emerging science of nursing based upon research gains stature and credibility, the doctor of philosophy in nursing degree will become the prestige degree in the future.[38]

It should be noted, however, that not all nurses with the Ph.D. degree have strong research backgrounds and that some nurses with doctorates other than the Ph.D. do have strong research backgrounds.

COMMUNICATION OF RESEARCH FINDINGS

Nurse scientists need to utilize as many means for the exchange of information as are available to them. All too often, research reported in nursing is somewhat old. However, with more research conferences, symposia information is transferred more rapidly. The use of newsletters and journals for transmission of information certainly cannot be overlooked. For example, the information for authors sheet in the journal *Research in Nursing and Health* has a note stating that an effort is made to notify prospective authors within four to six weeks about acceptance of their articles for publication. Computers and satellites for exchange of research have tremendous potential as added means of communication. The Nursing Child Assessment Satellite Training Project, in which Dr. Kathryn E. Barnard and Dr. Robert E. Hoehn serve as investigators, is an illustration of the ability to share the findings of research through continuing education for the purpose of improving practice. The originating site of the satellite program is the University of Washington in Seattle, with participating sites of various types in six eastern locations and six western locations. Satellite transmission of current research may result in asking ourselves the question, "Is dissemination so rapid that means of peer review will also need to be altered?"

Accurate predictions are probably not possible, but means for deriving reliable forecasts would at least allow more convincing communication, and permit some planning. Delphi and cross-impact analyses have acquired some prominence in analysis of the future. Helmer makes the following statement.

Standard operations—research techniques, in order to be applicable to the demands of future analysis, with its requirement for forecasting changed conditions of the future operating environment, have to be augmented by judgmental information. Delphi represents a useful communication device among a group of experts and thus facilitates the formation of a group judgment. Cross-impact analysis, by focusing systematically on the casual inter-relationships between potential future developments, seeks to establish the next best thing to a (non-existent) theory of such phenomena.[39]

Lindeman used the Delphi approach in identifying priorities for nursing research, as viewed by nurses who have different functional roles. Perhaps more studies using the Delphi and cross-impact analyses would aid the profession in planning for the future.

REALISM REGARDING FUNDING

Grants

The competition for research funds is high and is likely to continue.

The retrenchment of research funds during the past few years has heightened the competition for grants. Gone are the days when research grants went begging. Though grants make up the largest category of support provided by the National Institutes of Health (NIH) it is suspected that only about 50 to 60 percent of the applications are approved by merit review committees, as these applications must survive a strict priority valuation before actually being funded.

The Bureau of Health Manpower, Division of Nursing, Nursing Research Branch has had approved unfunded grants, following review, FY 1975, 1976, and 1977. Research dollars in health have for the most part been poured into categorical disease areas. Federal support for biomedical research, primarily through the NIH, is primarily based on charters. Consequently, research which deals with patient interactions with the environment, the promotion of health, and the prevention of disability and infirmity, in which nursing is interested, is for the most part—except for the Division of Nursing—without federal sources for funding in terms of research grants.

However, nurses who engage in research which may fit into the categories of the NIH and other federal agencies should submit their proposals. Of course, proposals submitted to any potential source need to be convincing and well written. They must demonstrate that the nurse scientist is a "good risk." Grant writing is an essential skill for investigators. If grants are disapproved, the nurse scientist, like other scientists, should try to find out why. It's no disgrace to have a proposal disapproved. It is important that the investigator understands the disapproval so that decisions regarding the proposal can be made. Federal agencies will provide a summary statement indicating reasons for disapproval. In most agencies, consultation with the staff regarding proposal ideas can be discussed prior to submission. Investigators should take full advantage of these opportunities. The research grant program is designed to support distinct research projects and, though the competition is high, well-prepared nurse scientists can compete.

There are three basic types of grants. The *Research Project Grant* is awarded to an institution on behalf of a principal investigator for the purpose of allowing the investigator to study a focused area of research. The *Research Development Grant* is designed to improve the research abilities of such units as colleges of nursing. Enhancement of the research climate and promotion of research activities can be fostered through development grants.

Research Program Project Grants are directed toward a range of problems with a central research focus or theme and are usually considered long-term research programs. These may have several projects. Research centers in nursing could attempt to establish definitive research programs. The research center notion is a positive one—one of its major advantages is the opportunity to conduct research in a defined area. The opportunity to study an area in all its various facets and to consider varying approaches makes the center approach even more attractive. These grants are awarded to the institution on behalf of a principal investigator. The nursing research centers at Wayne State, headed by Dr. Jean Johnson; at the University of Illinois, headed by Dr. Harriet Werley; and at Ohio State, headed by Dr. Jo Ann Stevenson, are three examples of centers that have been established within nursing colleges and universities.

Another source of funds for research through federal agencies is the *Research Contract.* It is awarded for specific research believed to be necessary for our society. Nurse scientists are able to compete for these funds. However, except through the Division of Nursing, chances of being principal investigators on contracts are slim because of the nature of the research. Opportunities to serve as a coprincipal investigator are more possible. Nurse scientists should have their names placed on the various mailing lists of the federal agencies for announcements regarding contracts and grants.

Foundations are another source of potential funds for nurse scientists. These could probably be utilized more. The money crunch for research endeavors forces nurse scientists, as well as other scientists, to present convincing proposals which merit funding. Companies involved in the production of goods and materials used in health care might also be approached. Most companies do have their own research and development areas, but if their products are used in research, or improvements in products are recommended on the basis of research, they should be willing to fund outside research. Book companies and food processing companies are also potential sources of funds, as are individuals. Acquaintance with the bankers in the community may be useful in making contact with people who are looking for worthwhile projects to support. Inventions by nurse scientists, now rare, are likely to increase in the patient care area as research activities increase.

Nurses are known to receive relatively low support for research. Is it because they do not apply for funds? Is there a trend more toward contracts and away from unsolicited research? Are the studies proposed by nurses seen as valuable to society? What is the success rate of proposals which are written by nurses? As funds are sought these and other questions need to be answered.

FEMALE SCIENTISTS

The advantages and disadvantages of being a scientist are briefly discussed. Although most nurse scientists are women, the frustrations of functioning in a male-oriented society should not deter their determination to contribute to society as scientists. Women scientists need to understand that most traditions, rules, and implicit codes are male-oriented. Learning the system, how organizations work, and how to manage in a culture which is male-dominated is probably more helpful than worrying about how things should be. A realistic view of how things are, deliberate planning of goals, and concentration on how these goals can possibly be reached within the system are likely to have a greater payoff than complaints and worry. More commitment to accomplishing set goals is essential if nurse scientists are to meet the challenge of contributing to the improvement of modern health care.

Women scientists do have some unique problems. Though many of them possess energy, talent, commitment, and high production, there is an exclusion from the informal channels of communication. The "old boy network" seems to operate and men are either indifferent to or unaware of their exclusion of women. White suggests that women in similar fields of interest can often profit by forming, or joining other women in, associations which provide professional stimulation and motivation, as well as information and access to new opportunities.[40] It would be helpful if every senior nurse scientist would make an effort to sponsor or be supportive to at least one junior nurse scientist in her area of expertise. It would also help to identify how women in other positions could be helpful to women scientists.

A women in foundations survey, 1976, revealed that women trustees of foundations represent 19 percent of trustees, a one percent gain since 1973. There are 1.52 women trustees per foundation, as opposed to 6.47 trustees per foundation. Twenty-nine percent of foundation professional staff members are women.[41] Information such as this may be useless, but it may also help women scientists realize that these women can be helpful to them when they seek foundation grants.

The emotional or family support that men with doctorates have is probably different from that of women with doctorates, since over 95 percent of the men are married in contrast to only 50 percent of the women. In a study by Simon and associates, practically all unmarried women Ph.D.s without children worked full time in the "practice of their trade." Sixty percent of the married women Ph.D.s with children worked fulltime and 25 percent of these women worked part time.[42]

LONG-RANGE PLANNING

Not enough can be said about the necessity and importance of planning for nursing research. Too often there is planning for the educational and service components but little or none for research. Definitive predictions about the future can never be anything but assumptions about alternative actions. Sound alternatives usually result from planning. The area of research administration has hardly been tapped in nursing. This writer sees it as a critical and important focus in nursing. The obsolescence of knowledge necessitates that nursing research assumes as prominent a role in the scheme of the profession as nursing service and nursing education.

Planning for research is important to the continuous revitalization of the knowledge base and the people in the profession.

CONCLUSION

Nurse scientists will need to be patient. Gortner notes that science in nursing is emerging slowly.[43] Though it is moving slowly, there are indicators that it is gaining momentum. There will continue to be dark or dim periods, but the overall future looks bright.

Nurse researchers must find ways to incorporate findings into practice. Castles notes it is the responsibility of the nurse investigator to validate the clinical "hunches" of her practitioner colleagues, but it is the responsibility of those colleagues to utilize the findings and to identify further research questions.[44] Research application is a must since much of the research that is done in nursing falls into the category of applied research. Stetler and Marram[45] have proposed a model for the utilization of research findings in nursing practice which may be useful for the practitioner. Using this new knowledge in the practice of nursing may be as exciting as solving problems through the use of the research process.

The scope of nursing knowledge and skill has grown tremendously and both nurses and others in society recognize this. However, the visibility of nursing as a profession in its own right still remains somewhat blurred. When society accepts the fact that nurses are health professionals in their own right, it will not be difficult to establish an Institute of Nursing, a Bureau of Nursing or even a Department of Nursing in the system of our government. The future holds the answer.

REFERENCES

1. L. Notter, "Nursing Research is Every Nurse's Business," *Nurs Outlook* 11 (January 1963): 49–51.
2. M. Hayes, "Nursing Research is Not Every Nurse's Business," *Can Nurse* 70 (October 1974): 16–18.
3. A. Jacox, "Nursing Research and the Clinician," *Nurs Outlook* 22 (June 1974): 382–85.
4. L. Notter, "The Case for Nursing Research," *Nurs Outlook* 23 (December 1975): 760–63.
5. Bureau of Health, Manpower, Division of Nursing, Announcement of Predoctoral and Postdoctoral Nurse Fellowship Program, National Research Service Award Act of 1974, amended by Title II of P.L. 94-278, March 1977. Bethesda, Md.: Health Resources Administration, 1977.
6. P. Abelson, "A Report from the Research Community," *Editorial Science* 194 (October 29, 1976): 194.
7. S. Gortner, "Research for a Practice Profession," *Nurs Res* 24 (May–June 1975): 193.
8. F. Abdellah, "Overview of Nursing Research, 1955–1968, Part I," *Nurs Res* 19 (January–February 1970): 6–17.
9. American Nurses' Association Commission on Nursing Research, *Science in Nursing: Toward a Science of Health Care,* Kansas City, Kan. (American Nurses' Association, 1976).
10. M. Leininger (ed.), *Nursing Research Support Center Newsletter,* October 2, 1975.
11. C. Lindeman, "Priorities in Clinical Nursing Research," *Nurs Outlook* 23 (November 1975): 693–98.
12. R. Schofeldt, Accountability: A Critical Dimension in Health Care, in Health Care Dimensions. In Leininger, M., ed., *Transculture Health Care Issues and Conditions* (Health Care Issues, Part I), (Philadelphia: Davis, 1976).
13. "Salk: Holistic Health Approach Inevitable in 'Epoch B.'" *Brain Mind Bull* 2 (Sept. 17, 1977): 1, 3.
14. M. Rogers, *An Introduction to the Theoretical Basis of Nursing* (Philadelphia: Davis, 1970).
15. E. Ubell, "Health Behavior Change: A Political Model," *Prev Med* 1 (March 1972): 209–21.
16. U.S. Department of Health, Education, and Welfare, *Forward Plan for Health.* FY 1978–1982 Washington, D.C.: USGPO, 1976.

17. L. Breslow and A. Somers, "The Lifetime Health Monitoring Program," *N Engl J Med* 296 (March 17, 1977): 601–8.
18. E. Ziegler, "The Unmet Needs of American Children," *Child Today* 5 (May–June 1976): 40.
19. E. Mullen, "Are Today's Children Becoming an Endangered Species?" *Foundation News* 25 (January–February 1977): 24–30.
20. D. Woodruff and J. Birren (eds.), *Aging: Scientific Perspectives and Social Issues* (New York: Van Nostrand, 1965).
21. Cambridge Research Institute, *Trends Affecting the U.S. Health Care System*. HEW Publication No. (HRA) 76-14503, Washington, D.C.: USGPO, 1976.
22. U.S. Department of Health, Education, and Welfare, National Center for Health Statistics, *Age Patterns in Medical Care, Illness and Disability, United States, 1968–1969*. HEW Publication No. (HSM) 72 1026 Washington, D.C.: USGPO, 1972.
23. H. Grace, *Commentary on the Proceedings of the Scientific Session in Primary Care by Nurses: Sphere of Responsibility and Accountability* (Kansas City, Mo.: American Academy of Nursing, 1976).
24. American Academy of Nursing, *Long-term Care in Perspective: Past, Present and Future Directions for Nursing* (Kansas City, Mo.: American Academy of Nursing, 1975).
25. U.S. Department of Commerce, Bureau of the Census, *Statistical Abstract of the U.S.* Table 128 (Washington, D.C.: USGPO, 1974).
26. *Ibid.*, Table 139.
27. U.S. Department of Health, Education, and Welfare, *Forward Plan for Health, FY 1978–1982* (Washington, D.C.: USGPO, 1976).
28. G. Blinick, E. Jeraz, and R. Wallach, "Methadone Maintenance, Pregnancy and Progeny," *JAMA* 225 (July 30, 1973): 477–79.
29. S. Cohen and W. Olson, "Drugs that Depress the Newborn Infant," *Pediatr Clin North Am* 17 (November 1970): 835–50.
30. C. Williams, "Nurse Practitioner Research: Some Neglected Issues," *Nurs Outlook* 23 (March 1975): 172–77.
31. S. Ketefian, "Application of Selected Nursing Research Findings into Nursing Practice: a Pilot Study," *Nurs Res* 24 (March/April 1975): 89–92.
32. S. Gortner, D. Bloch, and T. Phillips, "Contribution of Nursing Research in Patient Care," *J Nurs Admin* 6 (March–April 1976): 23–28.
33. American Nurses' Association, *Priorities for Research in Nursing* (Kansas City, Kan.: American Nurses' Association, 1975).
34. Committee on Government Operations, *Health Research and Training. The Administration of Grants and Awards by the National Institutes of Health*, Second Report, 87th Congress, House of Representatives, 1961.
35. F. Downs, "Doctoral Education in Nursing: Future Directions," *Nurs Outlook* 26 (January 1978): 56–61.
36. G. Andreoli, "The Status of Nursing in Academia," *Image* 9 (October 1977): 52–58.

37. H. Grace, *Study of Resources for Doctoral Education in the Midwest* (Evanston, Ill.: Committee on Institution Cooperation, 1976).
38. M. Pitel and J. Vian, "Analysis of Nurse-Doctorates," *Nurs Res* 24 (September–October 1975): 340–51.
39. O. Helmer, "Problems in Future Research," *Futures* 9 (February 1977): 18.
40. M. White, "Psychological and Social Barriers to Women in Science," *Science* 170 (October 1970); 413–16.
41. J. Oliver, "Women in Foundations are Challenging the Status Quo," *Foundation News* 17 (July–August 1976): 31.
42. R. Simon, S. Clark, and K. Galway, "The Woman Ph.D.: A Recent Profile," *Social Problems* 15 (Fall 1967): 221–36.
43. S. Gortner, "Scientific Accountability in Nursing," *Nurs Outlook* 22 (December 1975): 764–68.
44. M. Castles, "A Practitioner's Guide to Utilization of Research Findings," *J Obstet Gynecol Nurs* 4 (January–February 1975): 50–53.
45. C. Stetler and S. Marram, "Evaluating Research Findings for Applicability in Practice," *Nurs Outlook* 24 (September 1976): 559–63.

INDEX

A

Abdellah, F., 153
Abelson, P., 154
Abortion, 125, 126, 142–43
Abstract for Action, An, 20
Academic Degree Structures, 26
Academic settings, 4
  nurse doctorates in, 15
  nurse fellows in, 3
  nurse scientist trainees in, 3
Academic socialization, 34
Accreditation, 3, 19, 45
Ackerman, W., 78
Acute care settings, 7
Adaptation model, 93, 94, 96–97
Administrators, 54, 57, 58, 90
Aged
  long-term care and, 160
  need for research on, 158–59, 164
  as research subjects, 127, 130
  special services for, 7
  studies of, 5
Alcoholism, 72
  need for research on, 160–61
Alfidi, R., 111
Ambulatory clinics, 10, 11
American Academy of Nursing, 42,
  159, 160

American Association of Colleges of
  Nursing (AACN), 3, 45, 49, 51
American Cancer Society, 44, 64
American Heart Association, 44, 64
American Journal of Nursing, 13
American Journal of Nursing Company, 46, 150
American Nurses' Association
  Commission on Nursing Education,
  3, 34
  Commission on Nursing Research,
  2–3, 16, 42–43, 44, 50, 51,
  150–51, 154, 163–64
  Committee of Research and Studies, 16
  conventions, 2, 16
  Council of Nurse Researchers, 16,
  42, 44–45, 49, 50, 51, 151
  guidelines for protection of human
  subjects, 109, 111
  Health Services Administration, 8
  membership of, 149
  minority nurse research fellowship
  program, 152
  peer review committees, position
  on, 138
  quality assessment and, 8
  research conferences, 42
  research guidelines, 141, 142